LOOKING GOOD

MY PASSION FOR OPTOMETRY AND THE LIVES I'VE CHANGED

From Digital Screen Time and E-Sports to Macular Degeneration From Binocular Vision to Cataracts and Glaucoma And Everything In Between

DR. BOB ROTHBARD

ISBN: 978-1-7332550-4-2

DEDICATION

To my mother, Eleanor "Ellie" Rothbard. My mom was a gem of an individual. I was fortunate to have her as my neighbor in Rancho Cucamonga for fifteen years. She got along well with everyone and was loved by all who knew her. She passed on January 31, 2018, at the age of ninety-six.

My mother loved being with people. I am involved with a few of the Chambers of Commerce in my area, and I would take her to events that they put on. Her engagement with my friends and other members of the chambers was wonderful.

Ellie was also a bridge enthusiast. She played at the local senior center once or twice per week, even up until a few weeks before her passing. She was adored by her local bridge players.

When it came to family functions or just going out, her first response was always "Yes." What a wonderful attitude.

I was just watching a show which quoted Abraham Lincoln (I believe): "It's not the years in your life but the life in your years." This surely applied to Ellie.

Finally, I will quote Gary Vanynerchuk: "It's legacy versus currency." For my father, sister, her son-in-law, her grandson, great-grandchildren, and me, her legacy was second to nobody.

REVIEWS

"I never knew there were so many things that could happen with your eyes."

—Danielle Henderson, patient

"Dr. Rothbard's book contains a fascinating array of interesting patients. He is a master at telling the story of each patient in a brief easy to understand manner. It is obvious to me that Dr. Rothbard is an insightful optometrist who, thanks to the dedication to his craft, is highly gifted at problem-solving. His passion for his patients is abundantly evident. I recommend this book to those interested in vision and eye health. I also recommend it to those interested in how a skilled, caring, healer optometrist thinks his way through the excellent care of his patient."

—John "JT" Tassinari, OD

"A fascinating window into a long and productive life of an optometrist. The book is insightful about the profession's past, present, and future"

—Pinakin Davey OD, Ph.D., FAAO

Dr. Bob takes us through his journey through the eyes (and vision or lack thereof) of his patients. It is through the patient stories in this book that we get to know the

Optometrist, friend, colleague, and man that so many love and respect. His knowledge and caring heart are both evident when reading his book. He recognizes that his work is not over. He has generations to care for and he genuinely wants to help everyone. When you walk away from this read, you will be uplifted that there are some doctors that still care about the patient's well-being as opposed to the big business of insurance companies. From personal experience, the words in this book are factual. Kick back and enjoy the read. Let Dr. Bob show you kindness through his world.

—Amy Valdivia, patient

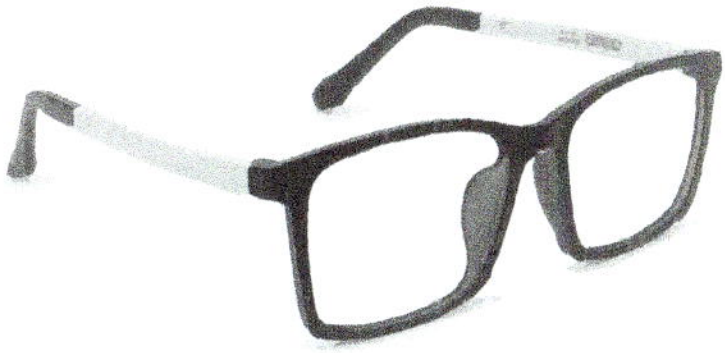

FOREWORD

"I wrote this book for individuals who might not realize what optometry is all about... individuals interested in becoming optometrists and optometrists themselves could benefit from reading this book." I would have to agree with Dr. Rothbard. He has a way of telling stories. Through his patient stories, written from the perspective of a doctor through the eyes of his patients, the reader can realize what optometry is all about—the diversity of patients whose lives can be changed and in some cases saved! Dr. Rothbard's in-person eye exams provide the opportunity for relationship building with his patients, something telemedicine can never replace. Dr. Rothbard is the epitome of a behavioral optometrist. He writes about the art of healing—the art and science of eye and vision care.

Dr. Rothbard's patients' stories illustrate the reasons why patients with eye problems seek their optometrist even before seeing their PCP. The portions of the manuscript on systemic diseases and how they manifest in the eye and vision system, with patients either coming in with symptoms or not, illustrates how the optometrist's findings during the course of an eye exam may diagnose a systemic problem such as diabetes or high cholesterol.

Dr. Rothbard is able to stay connected to the health professional doctor reader and the lay audience, balancing technicality and practicality throughout the book.

Dr. Rothbard's readers can be his future patients. Reading his book allows the reader to know who he is as a doctor. And for the optometry student, perhaps to see into the life of a private practice optometrist and what the practice of optometry holds.

Dr. Rothbard adds heart to optometry. Dr. Rothbard tells the story of influencing a gym staff to become an optometrist who graduated in 2015. I am certain this book will influence those who haven't considered optometry to consider this fabulous health profession and those who are already optometry students to further understand the depth and breadth of practicing optometry to its fullest. And for educators and practicing optometrists, this book is a wealth of patient stories to renew what we do, and how we change patients' lives every day. He reminds us that patients may not care what we have to say until they know the doctor cares.

—Ida Chung

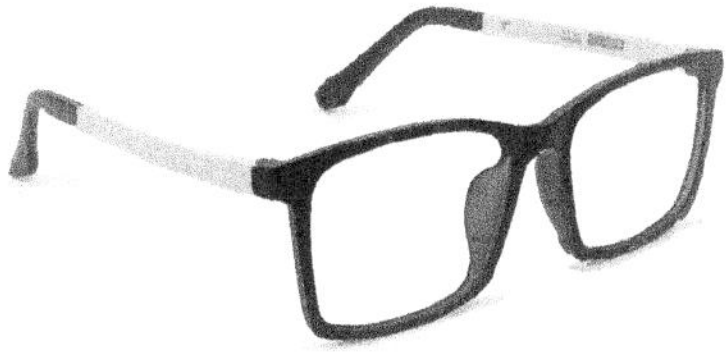

INTRODUCTION

Ever since my junior year in high school, I've wanted to become an optometrist. My book will span the years of my first applying to optometry school to my current state of practice. A major part of the book will describe some of my patients whose lives we impacted significantly. The book will briefly touch upon various conditions pertaining to the vision and the health of the eyes. I will also cover briefly some of the spectacular advancements that have occurred in the profession since I graduated in 1981.

My years in practice have been a wonderful journey, one that I wouldn't trade for anything. My passion and love for the profession should be evident from reading this book. Toward the end of the book, I'll direct you to areas on social media where you can find more specific areas of my career in optometry. A niche area of visual need I'll be touching on later is the population engaged in e-sports. The reason I am excited about this is because of the tremendous growth in this area and the extreme visual demands of this sport on its participants.

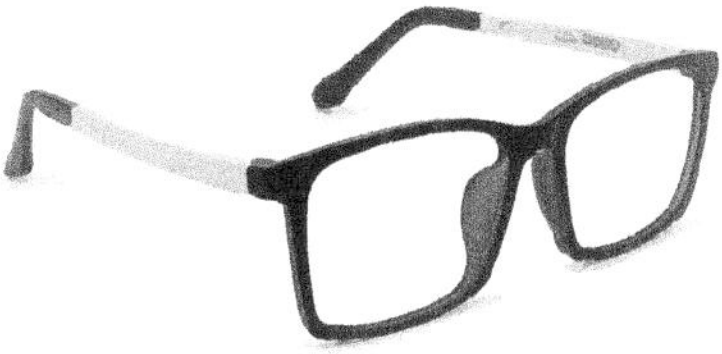

MY JOURNEY

I wanted to become an optometrist ever since my junior year of high school. I wanted something in the healthcare professions that was not life or death. Although in the course of my career, I would actually be involved with saving a couple of patients' lives. Also, optometrists made a relatively good income.

Academically, high school was never a problem. Undergraduate studies in Albany, New York, however, were difficult. I experienced the anxiety of having to get good grades so I could be accepted into optometry school. The competition was keen. In many of the required courses, called prerequisites, it didn't matter what you learned as long as you got a good grade. Many of the professors knew this. The stress was incredible. Many times I was up until eleven at night till one in the morning studying for a grade. That does not include some of the all-nighters I pulled before finals or midterms. I had about a 3.0 GPA which I knew was not good enough to enter optometry school. I realized early in my sophomore year that if I stayed in the current situation, I would never get into optometry school.

Right around this time, my mother suggested that I call a friend of the family (whom I'd never spoken to or met). He was currently attending optometry school in Oregon. It happened to be that his father was my parents' optometrist and his grandfather was my grandparents' optometrist. He told me that if I attended undergraduate school in Oregon, I would stand a better chance of getting into their graduate program in optometry. As a result of this call, I transferred out to Oregon the following year, did well in my junior year of undergraduate school and got accepted into optometry school. I dare say if I didn't make this call, chances are I wouldn't be an optometrist. And you know what, there are individuals who might not be alive today if I did not become an optometrist. I will describe one of those cases later in the book. Her name is Sheneen.

I was really focused (no pun intended) on getting into optometry. During my junior year of undergraduate, I took a preparatory course for the Optometry College Admission Test (OCAT). Despite a poor record with other standardized tests (especially the verbal scores), I did very well on the OCAT.

I applied for optometry school during my junior year. Digressing a bit, I thought it was interesting that one of the last courses I took to fulfill the humanities requirement to get into optometry school was Raku Workshop. This was a pottery course.

I knew when my application for optometry was being reviewed for consideration. The date the school reviewed a particular application was based on the state you were from. My application for the fall, 1977 class was being reviewed in early April. The following day the admissions director, whom I knew, asked me to come into his office. It was there that he congratulated me on being accepted into optometry school.

When I called my family and told them I was accepted, my father stated that was the best news he'd heard in years. It's hard to believe that I started with optometry school over forty years ago.

I feel so fortunate that I got to study at two optometry schools. I studied optometry for four years at Pacific University, College of Optometry. Different schools emphasize different areas of vision care. At the time, my school, Pacific University College of Optometry emphasized functional or behavioral optometry. In a nutshell, behavioral optometry emphasizes how what you do (for example sitting in front of any digital device) affects your vision. Behavioral optometry also deals with vision problems that can lead to learning problems. A third area of the relevance of behavioral optometry is how one's vision affects their performance in sports. Clarity, of course, is an issue, but hand-eye coordination, peripheral awareness, and depth perception are just as important in dealing with one's performance in a given sport.

Between my third and fourth years of optometry school, I attended the State College of Optometry in New York City for an internship in vision training and binocular vision. These two institutions helped shape the way I would examine patients and my thought that goes into diagnosing and treating them. Between the two schools and continuing education seminars, I would like to mention the names of a few of the professors and lecturers who helped shape the way I work with patients, all of who are optometrists: Beth Ballinger, Harold Haynes, Bill Ludlam, Nathan Flax, Martin Birnbaum, Elliott Forrest, Arnold Sherman, Jerry Sherman, Alan Cohen, Irv Suchoff, Jerry Getman, and Bob Sanet.

One of the most important sets of findings I obtained at school is how well the patient's eyes work together. Yes, it's important to have an individual see clearly out of each eye. After this, it's important to measure how well those two eyes work together. Most patients that I examine have straight eyes. In other words, their eyes align. A very important set of findings we obtain is how much effort it takes for those eyes to align and work together. I want to go into this a bit.

Basically there are two systems at work when it comes to discussing how well the eyes work together (binocularity). One is the aiming system, which tells you where the target is. The other system is the focusing system, which tells you what it is and if it's clear. For some patients, these systems work well together and for some, they do not. This is quite independent of whether the patient needs glasses to see clearly or not. Realize that after the age of forty the focusing system starts to break down. By fifty it is all but gone. I will discuss this more in-depth later.

I graduated from optometry school in 1981. I worked in different types of practice settings from 1981 until 1989 when I opened my practice, cold, after seven years of working for other doctors. A friend of mine who was an optician (an individual who assists in the fitting of glasses and contact lenses) convinced me to locate in an up-and-coming, developing area, Rancho Cucamonga, California. He came into the practice with me. We opened in a new strip center. I really enjoyed the doctoring part of the practice but was not good at the backend. After about three years, I was severely in debt. This situation lasted for several years. With time, however, things began to improve.

A bit of good fortune came our way. JP Morgan Chase wanted the area of the strip center where we opened twenty-three years earlier. As it turned out, they completely built me a new office to our specifications at basically no cost in another part of the same center. This was really a perfect way of upgrading one's practice. Also around this time, I was developing a staff that I was extremely comfortable to work with. The profits within the practice were growing. I am extremely happy with how the practice is doing now.

I feel so blessed that I chose optometry as my profession. I feel such a divine intervention in my professional relationships with my patients and colleagues. The impact that I've had on my patients' lives and the impact they've had on mine has been profound. I feel that the interest, empathy, and devotion I have developed for them over the years has helped shape my practice. I very strongly feel this way about the current staff I have with me. I would certainly say they're the main reason my practice is flourishing.

I was never a reader in my public school days. My SAT score on the verbal section the first time taken was 410. I probably had the lowest score in that category for anyone graduating from optometry school. Now I almost feel naked without a book. Most of the books I read deal with personal development. I'm going to start with my favorite. I believe this book should be part of the curriculum of every high school or junior high school. I also believe it has had a profound effect on my life. It was written in the mid-1930s. The name of the book is *How to Win Friends and Influence People* by Dale Carnegie. There was a lot of great information in this book. I believe the most important message delivered in the book and a central theme to it was how do you make someone feel important? If you can tap into this in a sincere way (not by flattery or "BS") you will improve your relationships with others and improve your own well-being in the process.

Social media over the last several years has had a really good effect on my practice. My assistant, Shelby, has helped me immensely with this. We're currently on Facebook, LinkedIn,

Instagram, Twitter, YouTube channel and Yelp. I have two Facebook Fanpages that deal directly with my business: www.facebook.com/ranchoeyedoctor and www.facebook.com/personallydevelopedself. My website is www.ranchoeyedoctor.com. On the website there are podcasts listed I've participated in with experts in our immediate area of California that deal with different areas of vision. I discussed areas of vision including LASIK, retinal disease, sports vision, vision training, systemic disease, especially diabetes and its effect on the eye, concussions and their effect on vision, and viewing digital devices and their effect on vision.

I am now celebrating being in my own practice for thirty years. It has been a great experience. I really don't see myself retiring. Paraphrasing that great movie: It's been a wonderful life.

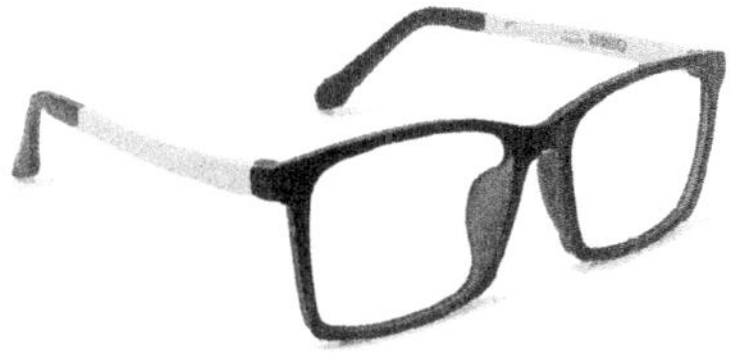

PART 1: MY PATIENTS

As stated, I've been practicing optometry since 1981. I have seen thousands of patients. In this section of the book, I will be discussing specific cases. Naturally, I cannot use real names and have changed both names and some identifying information of my patients. Even so, I hope you benefit from learning about these unique cases and that you can identify with some of these patients and their visual situations.

MARY

Mary was referred to my office about twenty years ago. Her chief complaint was that she was walking into walls after brain surgery. She couldn't walk straight. (I never found out why the patient had brain surgery.) This meant the patient couldn't drive, work, or even read. She was becoming severely depressed. What really was bad is that her surgeon was saying she was malingering, in other words, faking the symptoms. The examination revealed an extremely significant finding. First off the patient saw 20/20 in each eye. There was no glaucoma and the retina in each eye was normal. I did find, however, what was causing the patient's problem. When you measure a visual field, the patient looks straight ahead with one eye covered as flashing lights are presented. When we ran a visual field on each of Mary's eyes, measuring her peripheral vision, there was a glaring deficit.

Mary had a complete right-field hemianopsia. What the heck is that? When I covered the left eye with a patch, Mary could not see any flashes on the right side of her vision; she could only see the left side. When I patched the right eye, she was only able to see the flashes on the left side, nothing from the right side. This meant that if the patient was looking straight with both eyes open, she would not see anything on her right side. This is why she couldn't walk a straight line. This disruption of her visual world caused by the surgery led to all the symptoms she was suffering from.

How could the surgery lead to this problem? Visual fibers from each eye travel to the back of the brain to an area called the visual cortex. Depending on where the insult to the brain occurs via surgery, stroke, aneurysm, or tumor, a different visual field defect can occur. It is my guess that the surgeon cut the visual fibers leading to the above issue.

So what can we do? The fibers that had been cut could not be restored. Consequently, I prescribed prism for both eyes. Prism is a type of prescription that is incorporated into the lens that shifts the image up, down, left or right, depending on how they're held. I was able to put a prism in front of each eye that shifted the world to the left which helped her feel more balanced in her visual world. Afterward, she was able to walk in a straight line, read better, and her life was put back into order. What a great feeling for both the patient and me.

One last fact. Mary launched a malpractice suit against the doctor. It is important to realize that the doctor might not have committed malpractice. The surgery could have necessitated a cut of the visual fibers to alleviate the patient's neurological problems. If the surgeon would have run a visual field, he certainly would have found the underlying cause of the patient's problems that occurred after the surgery.

It's possible that if the doctor hadn't made the patient feel so insignificant and tell her she was faking the symptoms, maybe the suit wouldn't have occurred. A little empathy would have gone a long way. Empathy is significant in a healthcare environment

STAN

Stan was a long-time patient of mine. Stan was around sixty-three years old and had a history of glaucoma, which was more severe in the right eye. He lost most of his vision there and some of the peripheral vision in his left eye. Stan was very nearsighted with astigmatism in both eyes. He recently had cataract surgery in the right eye, which left him with some astigmatism. There was now a significant difference in prescription between the two eyes. We prescribed him a new pair of glasses, which gave him a lot of problems. This is because of the difference of prescription between the two eyes which led to different sizes of images for each eye. I then prescribed him a pair of contact lenses. His expression of happiness with his vision was worth its weight in gold. He said this was the first time in a long time he could see clearly and comfortably with good depth perception. Generally speaking, when a patient has a significant difference between the two eyes in prescription, glasses will lead to a difference in image size between the two eyes. However, when fitted with contact lenses, the image sizes for the two eyes will almost be the same, regardless of the difference in prescription. Reading was also good as he was able to use standard reading glasses for close-up and computer work. He was so excited—and so was I!

NANCY

Nancy came in complaining of blurred vision and eye fatigue. She was forty-four years old and worked about eight hours per day on a desktop computer. She was complaining of both far away and close up vision. Our findings showed she needed a different prescription for distance and near and a separate prescription for the computer. When we showed her the prescriptions, she saw a significant improvement.

One last thing. I found that Nancy's eyes did not line up vertically. I prescribed prism for this, and that also made a big difference for the patient. One of the complaints Nancy had was that she was very sensitive to sunlight, never going outside without sunglasses. When I took her outside and demonstrated the correction for the vertical misalignment (prism), her sensitivity to the light outdoors with both eyes open was significantly diminished. It was also interesting that when Nancy covered each eye separately (without any prism), there was no sensitivity to light. The fact that Nancy had trouble coordinating both eyes together led to her sensitivity to light. The prism also helped Nancy to see more clearly for distance and near. What's important, also, is that the misalignment of her eyes was extremely small, but still affected her significantly.

GAIL

Gail was originally seen in my office in 2018. She was a contact lens wearer with a fairly significant prescription. Gail had a problem in that her best-corrected vision in her left eye with either contact lenses or glasses was 20/70 and getting worse. I was able to see there was some pathology around the macula in the central portion of the retina in the back of the eye. The patient wanted me to give her a prescription for contact lenses, but I said I would not until she saw an ophthalmologist who could better determine what the condition of her eye was.

One year later, the patient came back into the office. She started out by reminding me that she was not happy that I hadn't given her a prescription for contact lenses and that I had her see a specialist first before I would release the prescription. She then stated she was thankful that I stood my ground. She wound up visiting the ophthalmologist and that doctor was determined she had a macula hole that required surgery immediately. She related to me that the surgeon stated that she could have lost her central vision in her eye if immediate treatment wasn't administered. I thanked Gail for telling me this story. Fortunately, everything worked out well. Even though Gail could not achieve 20/20 vision in that eye, the vision did not get any worse.

STACEY

I examined Stacey very recently in my office. Stacey was around fifty years old and had problems with both reading and distance. In a majority of these patients, I prescribe a bifocal so the patient can see distance and read with just one pair of glasses. This did not work well for Stacey. Every time she looked down through the bifocal she would get dizzy. This was whether she was wearing a lined bifocal or a progressive lens without a line. In Stacey's case, we had to prescribe one pair of glasses for distance and one pair for reading. This was quite inconvenient for her, but she didn't really have a choice. Sometimes contact lenses could really help to solve the problem, but in Stacey's case, she was not interested. We always discuss with the patient options that are available to them and the advantages of each. Generally, the patient has the final say on what they want.

JANICE

Janice came into the office with red eyes. She was a contact lens wearer. We prescribed medication which helped the problem. A couple of weeks later, after putting the contact lenses back in the eyes, they turned red again. Significant findings included a history of hypertension and not well-controlled diabetes. I was really concerned for her since when I looked at the back of her eyes, there was some bleeding of the retina present (not to be confused with the redness of the front of the eyes). It was imperative that Janice get her sugar under control. Diet and exercise were paramount. Janice also mentioned that she was under quite a bit of stress. Sometimes, eye problems are symptoms of something bigger. It is important to ask about a patient's life outside of their vision problems to get the full picture. Shows the importance of patient consultation and a patient-optometrist relationship

JUAN

This case dates back over thirty years.

I was working in my friend's practice at the time. A four-year-old boy walked into the practice with an outside prescription for glasses written by an ophthalmologist. The child was moderately far-sighted and his eyes tended to cross. Because of the prescription and the tendency for the eyes to cross, even with glasses, we tried fitting Juan with soft contact lenses. The eyes immediately became straight and he had full use of them. A few weeks later the mother returned to the office saying that her son was becoming very dizzy. Juan subsequently saw a neurologist whose diagnosis was that Juan had a cerebellar tumor. Upon removal of the tumor two very interesting findings occurred. The first was that Juan no longer needed any prescription for glasses. More importantly, Juan's eyes straightened without contact lenses. This case was most unusual. I shared it with my professional colleagues and they stated they had never heard of this type of case before. Even thirty years later, this case amazes me.

GENE

Gene has been a long-time patient in my office. He had a small defect in the macula of his left eye. Over the last few years, I have had trouble coming up with a glasses prescription for Gene. There are various reasons for this. Gene is now in his sixties. We finally got what both Gene and I thought was a good prescription. He came back about two months later stating that he had trouble seeing white letters against a dark background. He noticed some flare on the letters.

It was determined that there was some cataract formation, but keep in mind that the patient was corrected to nearly 20/20. Although there were cataracts, I wasn't sure this was causing the problem of flare. My big concern was that there weren't some changes in the retina, specifically the macula, the area of central, clearest vision. This case is ongoing. I referred Gene to a retinal specialist. I wanted to make sure there weren't any retinal problems before proceeding with cataract surgery.

I also want to mention something really important regarding cataract surgery for Gene if he does go through with it in the future. There are new intraocular lenses that correct for both far and near distances. Let's start out by saying (barring any problems with the retina) that most individuals who are corrected with the conventional type of intraocular lens (that corrects only distance) generally have great distance vision, but need reading glasses for up close. If a patient has worn contact lenses previously where one eye was corrected for distance and the other eye was corrected for near, the patient could have cataract surgery that mimics this. This is not a good idea for Gene as his left eye is was never totally correctable to clear 20/20.

The other way to give a patient both far and near vision is to prescribe multifocal intraocular lenses. The problem with these lenses, although they're getting a lot better, is that there is sometimes a compromise in the vision at a particular distance. Again, this would not be an ideal situation for Gene as his left eye will always have some blur due to the macula. Remember with Gene, I am now concerned whether there is blurred vision in the right eye due to the macula. Anyway, I told Gene if he goes through cataract surgery to please call me first.

JOAN

I get to feel pretty close to my patients. Joan came in for a routine examination as she turned forty-two and she was having problems with reading. Very normal. We got to talking and she was telling me about her husband looking to form a partnership with his boss in a business endeavor. She and her husband were Dave Ramsey fans and I Googled for her Dave Ramsey's opinions of business partnerships. For the most part, he was dead set against them. Joan recently came back to the office to pick up her glasses and she related to me that her husband wasn't interested any longer in forming the partnership.

What I really enjoy about optometry is that I get to know my patients and show an interest that they value and in some cases, I get to learn a thing or two from my patients.

↑ Author espresses his love for optometry as a patient-centred care

SHENEEN

Sheneen came in for an examination about six years ago. She entered complaining of blurred vision and headaches. These complaints are why many of my patients come in for an examination. When I looked at the back of the patient's eyes, I noticed that one of the optic nerve heads was blurry. This is quite abnormal. When we ran a visual field, there was a specific defect in each eye. The missing vision for each eye was identical. This indicates that the visual problem is due to something going on in the brain. We referred the patient immediately to an ophthalmologist. When the doctor conducted imaging tests of the brain, a very significant aneurysm was found. Surgery was immediately scheduled.

On the operating table, the aneurysm ruptured. Fortunately, the surgeon was able to save Sheneen's life; however, she did lose vision in one of her eyes. The surgeon told Sheneen that if she would have waited a couple of weeks longer, the aneurysm would have certainly ruptured and she would have died.

I've been following Sheneen yearly since the above episode. It's so rewarding to see her smiling face every year.

JACK

This is a very recent case. Jack came in contemplating contact lenses. Jack was about fifty-four years old. He was a competitive, amateur tennis player. Jack's vision at distance was relatively normal. He, like most fifty-four-year-old individuals, had problems with close-up vision. Recently, with technology improving with contact lenses, we fitted Jack with multifocal contact lenses. There's an expression that's sometimes used in healthcare (I did not invent it) that certainly applies to multifocal contact lenses: "Part science, part art, all heart." These lenses don't work on every patient but when they do, it's really great for the patient.

Multifocal contact lenses do not work like bifocal or progressive addition lenses for glasses. With glasses, you can only see close up by viewing through the bottom of the lenses. For example, if you were trying to view something close up on a store shelf at eye level or above with bifocal glasses on, you would have to tilt your head back to view the close-up print through the bottom of the lens.

Multifocal contact lenses do not work this way. It's as if you have simultaneous vision where you can see near or far without any head adjustment. Again, these lenses do not work on everybody but they're getting better all the time.

So what about Jack? I saw Jack on a follow-up visit to see how he was doing with his contact lenses. Jack said his friends were in awe. How he was playing so much better? They were wondering whether he had hired a professional coach. The reason Jack was able to play so much better (as related by him) was that the contact lenses he was fitted with helped him to see the spin on the ball and better tell where the ball was going to land. This is really crucial when it comes to superior tennis play.

MEGAN

Megan was an eleven-year-old girl who came in 2018 for an eye examination. She was only able to see about 20/80 in each eye. She was also unable to perform on the Ishihara color vision test and her peripheral vision was not good. Also of interest was the fact that even though she had some farsightedness, her vision without glasses should have been better. We did refer her to a specialist just to rule out any pathology. As it turned out, the specialist determined there wasn't any. The glasses we prescribed helped some. There was some improvement in her vision and peripheral vision, but it wasn't perfect. The patient and her mom related to me that her daughter was a cheerleader and that glasses would be a hindrance. At that time we fitted her with contact lenses. What a change. First off the patient's vision was a crisp 20/20 and her peripheral vision was normal as was her color vision. Most importantly for Megan, she was able to perform so much better in school and in cheerleading.

One possible reason for the above findings could be that Megan had a focusing system that was spasming. In other words, it didn't know how to relax. I have seen this before. This condition is called Streff Syndrome. Another patient, Jake, had a similar problem.

JAKE

Jake was an eight-year-old boy who came into the office complaining of blurred vision. His mother also stated that he was not doing well in school. When I examined Jake, I found his vision to be around 20/200 in each eye. What was interesting was that when I performed an objective test where I determine what the approximate prescription should be (without any input from the patient) I found the prescription to be very small. Ordinarily, this would not account for the patient's blurred vision. I also found that his color perception was off. I put the small prescription in front of Jake, and he was able to see a lot more clearly. Ordinarily, this low amount of prescription should have not made this big a difference in Jake's vision. Also, he was able to see the color charts perfectly.

Three things could account for this. The first possibility was that he was malingering—not being straightforward with us and just wanting to wear glasses. The second possibility was that there may have been some underlying neurological disease that needed to be ruled out. I did refer him to eye specialists, but he did not have any underlying issues. The third possibility, which I eventually gave as Jake's diagnosis was a spasming of the focusing (accommodative) system called Streff Syndrome. The focusing system could not relax and therefore he was unable to see clearly at any distance. When we prescribed a very low amount of plus prescription after ruling out any pathology from the professionals, there was an immediate positive result. We had Jake come back a couple of weeks after he received the glasses. His mother stated there was a huge difference in Jake's reading ability and he saw clearly at a distance.

Jake and his family moved away a few months after. About a year later, I got a call from South Carolina. As it turned out it was Jake's mother. The mother was inquiring what Jake's condition was. She wanted to tell Jake's current eye doctor what condition Jake had "that they don't teach much about anymore." I told her it was Streff Syndrome. I asked her how her son was doing and she said he was doing very well and had even improved in school.

eyesight improvement goes a long way

TOMMY

Tommy was an interesting patient. Tommy is fifty-three years old. Tommy has problems seeing clearly at a distance. In fact, it is marked on his driver's license that he needs glasses to drive. The problem is that all the glasses Tommy wears distort his world. In other words, everything he looks at is warped and the ground tends to rise towards him. This happens occasionally and especially for those patients who have astigmatism. There are reasons for this which I won't cover, except to say it has to do with the fact that the prescription is about a half an inch away from the eyes. With this in mind, I suggested to Tommy he try contact lenses. His first response was that he doubted he could wear them. I usually stop the discussion there about trying contacts, except I felt he had no choice. Since contact lenses sit on the eye there is a lot less distortion and warpage. I ended up fitting Tommy with one contact lens measured for distance and the other contact lens measured for near. If I fit both contact lenses measured for distance, Tommy would have not been able to read up close unless he used reading glasses over the contact lenses. Using one of each allowed him a lot more freedom and better vision. Needless to say, Tommy was quite happy with his vision.

LOU

Lou is a friend of mine. He works out at the gym with me and is sixty-eight years old. He knows he has cataracts and was complaining that he had trouble seeing, even with his glasses, especially at a distance. He told me his HMO stated his vision was not bad enough to have cataract surgery. Just a reminder, a cataract is a condition where the lens of the eye becomes cloudy and the individual, even with glasses, is not able to see clearly. I did not examine Lou. I asked Lou, "When you go out into brighter light, does your vision get worse?" He stated, "Definitely."

There are certain types of cataracts where the patient can see relatively clearly in normal lighting, but when they go into sunlight or look at bright lights their vision gets worse. One such cataract is called a posterior subcapsular cataract. The reason the patient sees worse with bright light is that the bright light causes the pupil to get smaller. With the position of the cataract in the lens of the eye and the smaller pupil, light has trouble reaching the back of the eye.

I told Lou to go back to the eye doctor and have them measure the vision with bright light off to the side that will cause the pupil to become smaller. If his vision is diminished to a certain level, he qualifies for cataract surgery.

As it turned out even after testing with the bright light. Lou's eye did not meet the criteria to have cataract surgery. However, it is possible that will change in the future and Lou can get the help he needs. Now, at least, they know what's wrong.

KATRINA

Katrina came into the office recently. Katrina was a medical school student who was nearsighted and really couldn't see clearly at a distance or near without glasses. As I described earlier, it is really important to measure how well a patient's eyes team together. Katrina's eyes were misaligned both vertically and horizontally. She was able to bring them together but it took a lot of effort. By prescribing prism in addition to her normal prescription, she told me it felt as if she was wearing no glasses. In other words, everything felt easy and natural.

One more finding that was important was that even though Katrina was twenty-five years old, she needed a different prescription for reading than for distance. Prescribing prism made a huge difference in her reading. Katrina never realized how much trouble she was having visually until we actually demonstrated the appropriate prescription. Once it was fixed, she actually had tears of happiness in her eyes.

JOANIE AND PETE

Joanie was a first-time patient when she was seen in my office. At forty-five years old, Joanie was an avid golfer—and had a big difference in prescription between her right eye and her left eye.

Joanie had worn progressive addition glasses but had never worn contact lenses. She found it very difficult to use her glasses while golfing. We discussed her options and decided to fit her with multifocal contact lenses. The results were amazing. First of all, her world jumped into 3-D as she was now able to use her eyes better together with the contact lenses as compared to glasses. Also, she was now able to focus clearly on the back of the golf ball. This helped her with her long game and particularly helped her with her putting. She told me she was now able to follow her ball in flight as she drove it (it's important to note that when the patients are in their forties or older if we prescribe for distance vision only, they'll have trouble seeing the back of the golf ball. That's why we prescribe multifocal contact lenses.) More important though was her putting game. When you're putting, you're actually about 3.5 to 4 feet away from the ball. As we get into our forties and older, it becomes increasingly difficult to focus between the golf ball and the pin. Since putting is really fifty percent of your golf score if you are a good player, this is really important. Joanie stated that as a result of wearing the contact lenses, she was now able to effectively focus her eyes between the back of the ball and the pin. She told me that her game improved immensely.

I have a good friend in Florida, Pete. Pete is in his early sixties and has been golfing for almost fifty years. Pete remarked that he was having increased trouble with reading the greens. Part of the reason for this is that he has trouble focusing from the back of the ball to the pin. Since I'm in California, I couldn't treat him. However, I did tell him about the multifocal contacts.

What's interesting is that Pete told me about his situation before I saw Joanie. Joanie allowed me to video her story about her improved golf performance as a result of the contact lenses and I subsequently sent the video to Pete. I told Pete to see an optometrist in his area who might be able to help him be fitted with these contact lenses. As of the writing of this book, Pete has not gotten the contact lenses. I feel if Pete were able to be examined by me, he would have gone through the fitting process for the contact lenses.

MICHAEL

Michael was a ten-year-old boy who entered the office in 2018. When I asked his father what his son's problem was, he felt that his son was suffering from "Alice in Wonderland Syndrome." I had never heard of this before. Of course, I Googled it. I found out its symptoms include the image going in and out of focus and perhaps getting bigger and smaller. Immediately I asked the kid how much digital work he was doing. He stated, "Sometimes when I am on my devices, I don't even blink." When we examined Michael I found that he likes to bring objects very close to read. I prescribed a mild prescription for close up which allowed him to view close up material at about 14-16 inches instead of the 6-8 inches at which he was viewing them. He felt he was able to see a lot more clearly.

There was a second problem with the patient that needed to be addressed. The patient, as well as his father, were significantly overweight. I told the father that for the welfare of his son as well as himself, they should go outside and exercise. Between relaxing his eyes and the stimulation of exercise, the patient should gain some relief from the above symptoms.

JASON

Jason was an introverted eight-year-old boy who came in for an eye examination. Jason had been seeing an ophthalmologist over the years for a lazy eye. The technical term for this is amblyopia. Jason's lazy eye was due to the fact that one of his eyes was perfect, had no prescription, and was easily able to see 20/20. Jason's other eye was about +5.00 and was only capable of seeing 20/100 with correction (glasses). Jason had undergone patching for years of the good eye to try to force the lazy eye to work. The best correction did not improve. A side note here. Amblyopia implies there is no pathology (disease) of the eye causing the best-corrected vision to be reduced. Since Jason was seeing an ophthalmologist over the years and I also examined his eyes, I was confident there wasn't any pathology.

When Jason came in, he was a bit withdrawn and quiet. His glasses made one eye look a lot more magnified than the other eye. I expected that this would cause him to see one image larger than the other. In most cases, the brain cannot take two different sized images and fuse them. What the brain does is take the blurred, magnified image and then suppress the image from that eye. If the brain does not do this, the patient sees double.

After I examined Jason, I went over the options for treatment with his parents. I strongly felt that Jason should be fitted for a contact lens in the lazy eye. When we placed the contact lens on Jason, there was an almost immediate response. He stated how much better his vision seemed. When he came back for a follow-up appointment, his parents stated how much more confident their son seemed. Over the next few months, they stated how his personality had become more outgoing. He actually wanted to go out for the little league.

Even though Jason was functioning a lot better, we were not able to improve his central clarity in the lazy eye. It is very important to note that there's more to good vision than just seeing 20/20. Jason was now able to use his eyes together as the image size for each eye was about the same. Also, Jason was able to observe a lot more peripheral vision on his left side when he was wearing the contact lens.

Over the years, Jason has come in for routine visual examinations. A couple of years ago, his father asked me to write a letter on behalf of Jason saying his visual situation was good enough to be allowed into the military. I crafted a letter on Jason's behalf. Jason was able to enter the military. I feel I could say that if we didn't fit Jason with the contact lens, his outcome in life would not have been the same.

A side note: Jason stopped by the office before I wrote this with his father to say goodbye as he was leaving for the military. He and his father extended their sincere thanks for being able to help Jason. It was really a wonderful feeling for me.

JEREMY AND DANIELLE

Jeremy came into the office complaining of blurred vision with his glasses. Blurred was an understatement. He was seeing 20/300 in each eye using his glasses. During the examination, he had mentioned that he was being followed by his previous eye doctor for keratoconus. Keratoconus is a progressive condition affecting the cornea. There is a misshaping and a thinning of the cornea. As this condition progresses, the patient is unable to see clearly with glasses. They can only see clearly with hard contact lenses. Sometimes the condition progresses to a point where they might actually need a corneal transplant. There is a new treatment for the cornea (which we'll discuss later) that keeps the cornea from deteriorating. I wound up referring Jeremy to a specialist for his condition. It takes a special type of contact lens to help the patient see clearly and I felt there were doctors more knowledgeable than I who would be better able to treat this patient.

I made a video about Jeremy and posted it on social media. I was back in The Bronx and I got a Facebook Messenger alert from Diane, a friend of my sister. I thought she was just sending me a Merry Christmas message. When I looked at the message she told me that she saw my video regarding keratoconus on

Facebook. She stated that her daughter, Danielle, was diagnosed with keratoconus. As a very concerned mother, she wanted to ask me specific questions regarding her daughter's condition. I was able to give her information regarding her daughter's condition and specialists who could help. I had discussed a relatively new procedure called corneal crosslinking. This procedure helps to strengthen the cornea and actually helps to improve one's vision.

A few weeks later, Diane told me her daughter followed up with a corneal specialist and had the procedure stating Danielle's vision had significantly improved. Subsequently, six months later, Danielle and Diane joined my sister, Martha, and me for dinner in Brooklyn. Danielle, who seemed incredibly happy, described how much better she was seeing. The power of social media sometimes is really great.

MARIE

The following is a story about an individual who was not my patient. I was at the 2018 Social Media Marketing World Conference in San Diego. After the meeting, I went to get a bite to eat. I was wearing my name badge indicating I was an optometrist. I got into a discussion with a lady who started telling me about her daughter. She said her daughter had a lazy eye. In questioning her fully, she described her daughter as having amblyopia. She was being patched, but her daughter refused to wear the patch. Instead, the daughter only wore her glasses. When I asked the mother, she said that one of her daughter's eyes looked a lot larger than the other one through the glasses. I told her that in most cases, it would be a lot better if her daughter could be fit with contact lenses.

As described earlier, when a patient comes in with a big difference in prescription between the two eyes, contacts should be recommended. In fact, some insurance companies would call these contact lenses "medically necessary." This designation pays a higher benefit. The patient with the lazy eye has a better chance for the two eyes to team together with the contacts. Afterward, the patient can undergo binocular vision therapy to get the lazy eye to see better and secondly have the two eyes function together.

The mother was from Maryland. She asked if her daughter could come out to California and be seen by me. I told her there were probably optometrists in her area who could take care of her daughter very well. I also told her that there is a group of optometrists who are Fellows in the College of Optometrists in Vision Development (FCOVD). She could actually call the phone number and get the name of a doctor. I also told her to share the conversation we had concerning her daughter with her daughter's eye doctor. I'm not sure what happened to Marie or her daughter, but based on Marie's enthusiasm, I can safely guess her daughter got the care she needed.

SAL

Sal has been a patient of mine for nearly twenty-five years. Sal has a prosthetic left eye. Anyone who only has one functioning eye should always wear glasses made of polycarbonate lenses for protection, even if they could see perfectly with the functioning eye. Sal related the story that he walked into a pipe that had struck his glasses. The lens did not shatter. It would have struck the prosthetic eye if he weren't wearing his glasses. Sal related to me what would have happened if he weren't wearing any glasses and the pipe struck his good eye. He said he could have done some severe damage to the eye. Again, keep in mind that the pipe might have shattered the lens if it weren't made of polycarbonate. Sometimes glasses don't just enhance vision, but protect it, too.

DEAN

Dean has a similar story. When I was going over lens options with Dean after his examination, I suggested to him that he wear polycarbonate lenses. He emphatically agreed. I asked him why he was so emphatic. He stated to me that when he was on the golf course, he got hit with a golf ball. He related to me that as he was trying to pitch out of the sand trap the ball hit the lip of the trap, ricocheted back and struck the glasses he was wearing which were fitted with polycarbonate lenses. He stated the ball actually dislodged the lens from the frame but the lens did not shatter. This episode probably saved Dean from the loss of vision in that eye.

MIKE

Mike came into the office about twenty years ago. Mike was in his early forties and applying for a position with the city. Because of the visual demands of the job, I had to clear him by saying he was visually able to perform his job. What's important to know is that Mike's best visual acuity with glasses or contact lenses in his left eye is 20/200. The right eye is 20/20. We fit Mike with a contact lens in the left eye. He was still only 20/200 but did have some depth perception. What's really important is that Mike has full peripheral vision in both of his eyes.

The city was reluctant to hire Mike due to his vision in his left eye. Mike went over with me the demands of his job. I saw no problem with him being able to perform them. I wrote a letter to the city saying Mike, visually, was a good candidate. A couple of weeks later, Mike informed me that he was hired for the position. Mike has come in for his vision care over the years and it has now been twenty years that he has been working for the city. This is truly rewarding for me as a doctor. This is one example of the ways that we have been able to change the lives of our patients.

KEN

Sometimes when we're working with patients, conducting a thorough exam, the glasses come back and the patient can't see clearly out of them. There are several potential reasons for this. The patient could have cataracts, macular degeneration, or a host of other pathological problems. The problem with Ken was something very different. He had dry eyes and they were irritated at times. Upon examination, the dry eye was not immediately noticed.

I administered a drop that helped with the situation called Pazeo. Pazeo is a combination drop that contains an antihistamine and a chemical that's called a mast cell stabilizer. There are cells in the eyes called mast cells. When they degranulate, they release a whole host of irritants into the eye. I've given this drop to patients in various situations and the results for some of them are amazing. When used on the appropriate patient, the result is almost immediate and it lasts up to twenty-four hours.

When I administered the drop to Ken, the results were really good. He was very consistent with his answers as to what he was seeing during the examination, which led to a really good outcome. Now when Ken comes in for an examination, he makes sure that he puts a drop in his eye the night before. Pazeo also drastically helped another patient named Amy.

AMY

I met Amy at a breakfast meeting at the local chamber of commerce. We introduced ourselves and I told her I was an optometrist. She proceeded to tell me that she suffered from dry eye and at times it was quite incapacitating. Some of this will sound similar to Ken's case above. She previously had refractive surgery which could cause a dry eye condition to become worse. No drops nor procedures would help. I invited her to come to my office and suggested Pazeo, the drop that helps those who suffer from irritated, dry eyes. The good thing about this drop is that it does not sting and you know whether it's going to work within a few minutes. As stated earlier, there is a dual mechanism for the way this drop works. It is an antihistamine and a mast cell stabilizer. The antihistamine works to dry the eye out while the mast cell stabilizer performs a different function. As stated earlier there are mast cells within the eye. When they break apart or degranulate, they release a whole host of irritants into the eye. Pazeo keeps the mast cells from degranulating.

Amy came into the office that afternoon. The results were great. She felt immediate relief from the drop. More importantly, when I called her the next day, her eyes were still feeling great. I scheduled Amy for a full examination to make sure everything else was normal with her eyes and found that otherwise, they were fine.

Amy was already seeing an ophthalmologist. She told me that he would write her a continuous prescription for the drops. I see Amy fairly regularly through network meetings and she states how her life has changed as a result of using Pazeo.

It's important to note that there is no one drop that's correct for everyone. That being said, I feel this drop has worked wonders for many of my patients and it's relatively safe.

DR. MARIA

Dr. Maria was a forty-six-year-old surgeon who was hoping to see more clearly with LASIK laser surgery. She had problems seeing distance and near, though her distant vision was not that bad. The problem with doing LASIK for Dr. Maria was that for her to see distance and near at the same time without glasses, they would have to create a situation where one eye was corrected for distance and one eye corrected for near. Since Dr. Maria had to have extremely precise vision for her to perform her surgery, this mode of correction was not acceptable.

I asked Dr. Maria if she wanted to try multifocal contact lenses instead, and she agreed to try them. She also got a pair of progressive spectacles when she wasn't wearing her contact lenses.

I promote LASIK wholeheartedly, but only in the right situation. It has made a tremendous difference for many patients. In Dr. Maria's situation, however, I felt LASIK was not in the

Doesn't force it and provides alternatives, broadening patient choice patient's best interest. It took a couple of trial pairs of contact lenses to get the best prescription but once she did, she was ecstatic about her vision, both far and near.

JILL

Jill entered the office wanting to wear contact lenses. Jill was seeing another doctor and complained of irritated eyes from her contacts. Her doctor referred her to specialists to see if there was a reason for this. This situation went on for a while. She subsequently came into my office for an examination and contact lenses. She told me about the above experiences she had with her contacts. From experience, I have had patients whose eyes were irritated due to having an allergic reaction to the contact lens solutions. This certainly was the case with Jill. When we switched the solutions, her eyes immediately felt better. It seems 2-3 percent of patients are allergic to some type of contact lens solution. Even though there could be many reasons for irritated eyes from contact lenses, this reason needs to be ruled out.

As a side note to this story, I just had a patient who stated they were allergic to the material of a specific contact lens itself. This is very rare.

WILL

Will was a first-time patient who complained of a sudden shift in his prescription. Will was forty-five years old and had always worn glasses to see clearly at distance. Over a few days time, he noticed that he could see really well at distance without any prescription. Was this good news for the patient? Unfortunately, in this case, the answer was no. The patient was also constantly hungry and thirsty. I referred Will to his primary care physician even before I examined him. My suspicions were confirmed. The patient's blood sugar was very high. He was suffering from diabetes. His physician put him on oral medications for diabetes and got his sugar under control. As this happened, Will's prescription reverted back to the same prescription he had before the onset of diabetes. Unfortunately, Will's prescription reverted back slowly. He could no longer see clearly without glasses at distance but his glasses prescription was still too strong.

I have found the best way to treat patients with fluctuating prescriptions is to fit them with disposable contact lenses. This way we were able to manage the change on a much more frequent and economical basis, as opposed to constantly changing the spectacle prescription. Eventually, with the normalization of Will's sugar over the next six weeks, we were able to prescribe Will with appropriate spectacles.

BILLY

I just saw Billy recently. Billy represents a type of patient for whom it is very difficult to give a glasses prescription. Billy had refractive surgery around twenty-five years ago, radial keratotomy. This was the type of surgery where the doctor placed incisions in the cornea of the eye. It was a fairly inexact surgery, especially as compared to the refractive surgeries like LASIK performed today. This surgery was mostly performed on patients who were nearsighted.

I have seen these patients come through the office over the years. The problem with this surgery is that many of these patients became farsighted and begin having problems with both reading and distance. When this surgery is performed, the cornea is weakened. Consequently, the shape of the cornea could change as a result of the pressure of the eye or other reasons that I cannot account for. What's important to realize is that the pressure of the eye changes throughout the day. With radial keratotomy, there are varying amounts of cuts made into the eye depending on the patients' refractive error (prescription). The more cuts the weaker the cornea becomes and the more subject to change the prescription becomes based on the change of pressure in the eye.

I have seen patients who have had radial keratotomy performed whose prescription fluctuates during the course of the day. This, of course, leads to a difficult task in prescribing for these patients. Additionally, due to the distortion of the cornea that is a result of the surgery, it is difficult to correct these patients with glasses to 20/20.

Billy came into the office having had radial keratotomy. I was able to derive a prescription for glasses that corrected him to only 20/30, fair but not great. Also, the prescription was fairly significant and there was a large difference between the two eyes. Every time I would show Billy the prescription, he would say it seemed clear, then a minute later, he would say it was no longer clear. Billy already had a pair of glasses which he said he no longer wore. The correction in these glasses was not very different from what I found. I spent a lot of time with Billy trying to come up with a prescription that would help him. Unfortunately, there was no ideal prescription that would help Billy. The good news is that I am seeing fewer of these cases as radial keratotomy has not been performed on a regular basis for over twenty years.

HEATHER AND JACOB

These cases are interesting in which they both came in back to back saying they lost their contact lens in their eyes. The first patient, Heather, had a decentered lens within her eye. Actually she had two lenses in her eye that were unaccounted for. It was actually easily seen with the biomicroscope. This was pretty straight forward.

Jacob's case was more interesting and a bit challenging. There was no lens in the patient's eye. However, there was a lash that actually starting growing and embedding itself into Jacob's peripheral cornea. I had to use an instrument to actually scrape the surface of the cornea to get the lash out. This, of course, is done with topical anesthetic. We then administered antibiotics to prevent infection. Everything turned out well.

JANET

Janet was a very recent case. In addition to having a cataract in the left eye, Janet had surgery for a detached retina that left her with double vision. This is not that unusual. The retinal surgeon had referred her to our office. At this time, Janet was wearing glasses that totally blocked the vision of her left eye so she wouldn't see double.

When I examined Janet, I found a very significant amount of prism for the left eye. If I were to put this amount of prism directly into the lens to alleviate the double vision, it would be incredibly thick. In this case, we used what's called a Fresnel prism which is actually a thin piece of plastic that adheres to the lens. This prism does diminish the clarity of what the patient sees.

When Janet received her glasses, she was still seeing a little double vision, but it was much better than it was. She stated when she twisted (torqued) the glasses just a bit, she would no longer see double. We saw how much and in what direction Janet had to twist the glasses and had the lab reapply the Fresnel prism.

When she picked up the glasses a second time, she was elated to find that she no longer had double vision.

MELANIE

Melanie came into my office a short time ago. She came into my office on an emergency basis with her friend. She was in tears due to pain. When I first examined her she could barely open her eyes and was extremely sensitive to light. Melanie was a contact lens wearer. The lenses were not in her eyes when she came in. She had taken them out. Melanie's condition was called superficial punctate keratitis, an inflammation of the front surface of the cornea. You can actually Google this condition and see what it looks like. Something had contaminated the contact lenses and caused this condition. I administered some medication that quieted the situation and made her somewhat more comfortable. I then told her to use unpreserved artificial tears every hour and come back tomorrow.

When she returned the next morning the eyes were completely healed. She literally said, "You really saved my life."

I said, "Not really."

She said she was having panic attacks and was depressed and was fearful she was losing her sight. It was great to see her smile in the office.

MARTHA

The following story is about a close relative of mine. Martha has been coming to me for quite a few years. She actually visits me from the East Coast. I tell her each year that her eyes need to be dilated. However, at her most recent visit, when I looked at a certain structure of the eye, I was concerned that if I dilated her eyes, the pressure in her eyes would rise significantly. I was also concerned about the small possibility that the pressure could rise if in a dark environment. This is called having a "narrow angle," which could lead to closed-angle glaucoma.

Closed-angle glaucoma is a dangerous condition since the high pressure could cause damage to the nerves of the eye and this could cause a loss of vision. The symptoms of this include severe headaches and nausea.

I referred Martha to an ophthalmologist. He thought the situation with her eyes was risky enough that they performed a laser procedure on a structure of the eye (iris) to keep a sudden rise in pressure from ever occurring.

Closed-angle glaucoma is relatively rare. I have referred only a handful of patients with this condition over my thirty years of practice to a specialist.

MARTY

Marty was a forty-four-year-old patient who came into the office complaining that he failed his vision test at the DMV. Marty had blurred vision at distance and close-up. He explained that he was involved with a video game that he purchased for an extreme amount of money, and he was in competition with other individuals around the world who were also playing it. He told me he was viewing his iPad for at least eight hours a day and foregoing any social contact. This certainly affected his vision.

When I showed him his prescription that he needed to see clearly, he was amazed by how clear his vision was. I certainly believe that all this close up activity affected his vision.

What's interesting to realize is how many individuals, especially kids, are involved with these games. Just look at Twitch and the whole area of Esports. The competition is intense. There is a lot optometry can do to improve upon the visual impact this intense amount of close up activity causes.

Most likely these individuals are not going to give up on their games. What's interesting is that through appropriate lenses and vision training we can actually improve upon the vision and performance of these "players."

Realize, however, that not all optometrists nor ophthalmologists are trained or subspecialize in this area of prescribing for near or vision training. The niche for this type of vision care is growing immensely and there aren't yet enough doctors working in it.

HANK

I met Hank at the 2019 E3 Conference in Los Angeles. This is a conference that deals with video games and Esports. Hank was a twenty-year-old student at Rensselaer Polytechnic Institute near Albany, N.Y. Hank was a developer of video games and was an active player. I told him I was an optometrist and he explained to me that he had a big difference in prescription between the two eyes and had to wear a contact lens in one of them. The other eye did not require any prescription. Many times when an individual has a big difference between the two eyes, their eyes have trouble working together. I had actually brought some low-powered lenses to the show and tried them with Hank.

I held some reading material about sixteen inches in front of Hank. I had him first read the material without the lenses and then had him read it while placing the lenses I'd brought in front of it. He felt a lot more comfortable reading the material at sixteen inches with the lenses. Of course, these lenses blurred his vision when looking far away. I told him when he goes back to N.Y., to contact his eye doctor and relay the information I shared with him. I really believe that his ability to view any digital device and play video games will significantly improve with lenses such as these.

LEE

I just examined Lee today (June 14, 2019). Lee worked in HR at her work viewing a monitor for several hours a day. Lee is around thirty years old and has worn glasses for distance. As I was completing the examination, Lee explained to me that as she was viewing the monitor wearing her glasses, she would have to get closer to it as her eyes started to blur. Many times on an individual younger than thirty-five, the prescription for distance is the same as the prescription for near. This wasn't the case for Lee. I held a pair of lenses in front of Lee over her distance prescription and had her view a monitor. She felt her eyes relax and she didn't have to sit so closely to the monitor.

Each patient is different. In the cases of Hank and Lee, these "near lenses" helped significantly. In other patients, they do not. Each patient has to have their near vision evaluated to see if these lenses could benefit them or if they'll make no difference at all.

MICHELLE

I recently received this direct message from Michelle as a result of an Instagram post. I was thrilled to receive it.

"Dear Dr. Rothbard!

My name is Michelle. I have been a PC gamer since I was in 3rd grade. I mainly play Overwatch and World of Warcraft. My friends and I are into competitive gaming. We practice every night. I have to wear glasses to play games though!

I admire your work. I find it fascinating and cool that a doctor is genuinely interested in E-Sports. A lot of gamers like myself strain our eyes."

I am enthusiastic about this tremendous niche for optometry and that gamers are reaching out. I sincerely feel I can help them with their visual needs, if not directly by treating them, then my giving them information on how to seek out appropriate vision care that can help them.

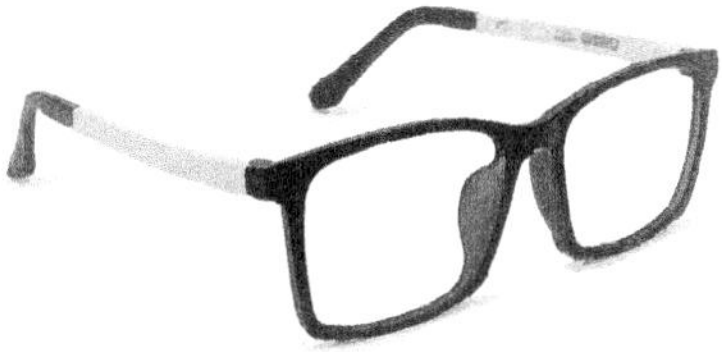

PART 2

Patient care involves everything from prescribing spectacles to consulting with surgeons. In this section, I'll be going into detail about the findings I take, the interpretation of the findings, and the discussion and treatment we deliver to the patient.

COMPREHENSIVE EXAMINATION

Case History. One of the first and most important findings we take during an examination is the case history. I want to know why the patient is there. Is the patient suffering from blurred vision, headaches, or are their eyes tired? I want to know whether their vision is getting worse. We also need to know what kind of work they're doing and, if they're a student, how well they're doing in school. I want to know if there are any medical conditions.

Vision. I then want to know what the patient is seeing, both with glasses (if they have them) and without glasses. This will give me information about whether or not the patient's vision is changing.

Examination. I then proceed to start the examination. I first start with an objective finding as to what the prescription is. "Objective" means I determine what the prescription is without asking the patient.

I then go through a battery of questions for the patient (the old familiar "which is better, one or two?") to get the clearest vision. From there we now want to measure how well the eyes team together. To put it simply, this part of the examination works with the alignment of the eyes, both vertically and horizontally, and at distance and near. I often find that when I perform this part of the examination, the patient says they never had these findings measured before. I will tell you right here that the precise measurement for prescribing these findings could be paramount. I have had many patients who can see clearly with each eye separately, but when both eyes are open, the patient feels uncomfortable looking through the glasses or contact lenses if these alignment findings are not taken into account. Also, we need to take into account if the prescription for distance is the same as the prescription for near. It is extremely critical to measure the findings up close for all patients, regardless of age. This is a finding that often gets overlooked by some doctors.

Another finding that is extremely important no matter what age, is to see if the eyes align differently at reading and distance. I have examined patients whose eyes are aligned perfectly at a distance while they seem to either cross or go apart at near. Some further findings I am interested in, depending on the type of demand or situation a patient places on their eyes, is how much stress I can put on the patients' eyes and still have them maintain a single (not double), clear comfortable vision. These situations could include spending extreme amounts of time doing close up work whether on the printed page or digitally. Also, patients who are extremely competitive in sports could have their performance affected by these stress findings. I will cover this more in-depth as I discuss sports vision and computer-related vision problems.

After I have gathered these findings, I then check the patient for the health of the eye. Using instruments I check the anterior and posterior areas of the eye. I also check the pressure within the eye. A very important finding is to check for the peripheral vision of each eye. To do so, we perform a visual field test. With one eye patched the patient looks at a central target and flashes of light occur off to the periphery. The patient then signals with a clicker when they see each flash of light. Abnormal findings with the visual field could indicate problems within the eye itself or the brain. Diseases of the eye can very much affect how well the patient is able to see through the prescription. Dry eye, cataracts, glaucoma, and macular degeneration are just four of many conditions that could prevent a patient from seeing optimally through a pair of spectacles or contact lenses. Some of these diseases will be discussed subsequently.

When we've obtained our findings, we then discuss with the patient what the best solution for their visual situation(s) is. Generally speaking, the solutions come in one of four forms: spectacles, contact lenses, surgery, and possibly vision training.

SPECTACLES

Spectacles (glasses), of course, come in many forms: single vision, lined bifocals, progressive addition lenses. The glasses need to match the situation the patient is using them for. There are two very important types of cases I want to discuss.

The first type of case is the child or young adult who performs a lot of close up work. Conventional thinking usually dictates with these individuals that the prescription for distance is the same as it is for near. A lot of times it is not. The problem is that the child might be able to see clearly at near through the distance prescription. However, the child could actually be straining their eyes to see. Also regarding children, they might be able to see perfectly at distance without glasses but need them for close up.

One finding I feel is paramount in prescribing for young individuals is how far they like to hold their reading material. If a young individual sees perfectly at distance with or without correction but likes to bring the reading material very close to see it, this patient might benefit from bifocals or just glasses that are meant for reading. I have found this finding in itself has made a very big difference for the performance of kids in school and individuals who are performing on digital devices, especially monitors.

Most of my adult patients perform much of their near work on digital devices. Desktops, laptops, cell phones, and iPads certainly fall under this category. I really feel the niche for optometry dealing with near vision is growing exponentially and the number of doctors trained to deal with the situation is not nearly keeping up.

I have a monitor set up in my exam room. I use it to help me prescribe my patients. When a patient tells me they work several hours a day on a desktop computer, I have them sit in front of my monitor to gauge how far they sit from the screen.

As an eye doctor, one must consider several factors. The first one is the age of the patient. It's really obvious that as a patient approaches their forties, their ability to focus up close diminishes. Some nearsighted patients might have blurred vision at distance but their near vision is good.

The first type of patient I want to discuss is the patient thirty-five and under who is performing on a desktop or laptop computer. Generally, these patients should have the same prescription for distance as compared to near. As stated earlier, when conducting a visual examination, no matter what the patient's age, in addition to measuring a patient's eye health and correction for distance, the doctor also needs to measure if the prescription for distance is the same as the prescription for reading and how well the eyes team together at those distances.

It's too often thought that on patients under thirty-five, that the prescription for reading and distance is the same. In many cases, it is not. Even with youngsters, we often find that even though they have no prescription for distance, they may indeed need glasses for near, especially if we notice that the patient brings the reading material inordinately close to read. There are ways to determine what the prescription should be up close but the most important thing is to actually show the patient what they'll see with the prescription as they're viewing the computer.

The patients who are in their forties and older almost always need a different prescription for reading as compared to distance. Several factors are very important to consider. The issue of a laptop versus desktop monitors is very important. In most cases, if the patient is using only a laptop or an iPad, the same prescription usually in the form of a bifocal for normal reading can be used for these digital devices. This is because they're positioned fairly close to the same distance and height as books or magazines.

The desktop computer poses a significant added consideration. The height of the screen oftentimes is at eye level. When a patient is prescribed a bifocal for everyday use, it's generally for distance and reading and the reading area is located at the lower part of the lens. If you're viewing a desktop monitor, generally it is located at eye level. Not only that but generally the monitor is located about twenty-four to thirty inches away. Oftentimes, a second bifocal (or progressive addition lens) needs to be prescribed for the workstation. If a patient uses a bifocal prescribed for distance and reading and tries to use it on a desktop computer, the patient will often have to tilt their head back to have their eyes positioned in the reading area of the bifocal and lean into the screen so they're at the appropriate reading distance for that pair of glasses.

What's appropriate is to prescribe a bifocal where the top part is measured for the distance at which the patient is viewing the monitor. The bottom part is measured for where the patient generally views text. The patient needs to know that this type of lens design will blur distance viewing. It's interesting that some patients don't need this second pair of glasses and that they're able to view everything with just one pair of glasses.

Another interesting factor regarding digital devices is the blue light coming off. Some of the devices have ways of filtering the blue light. Also, there are coatings that you can add to the lenses that help filter this blue light. Blue light is meant to simulate daylight. Consequently, if you view various devices emitting blue light, this could simulate daytime, suppressing melatonin within the body, and could keep one from sleeping. Also, there is some information that this blue light can possibly affect the macula of the eye, which plays the role of how well an individual is best able to see. If the macula becomes impaired, whether or not the patient wears glasses or contact lenses, they will not be able to see clearly.

CONTACT LENSES

The second main option a patient may choose to correct their vision is contact lenses. In my opinion, when contact lenses are appropriately prescribed, the vision is a lot more natural for the patient with less distortion. In general, the stronger the prescription, the more appropriate the contact lenses are for the patient. Also, if there's a big difference between the two eyes, contact lenses are significantly better for the patient. The reason for this is that when there's a big difference between the eyes and glasses are prescribed, the patient will be viewing two different size images. The brain will have a tough time bringing these two images together. This possibly could lead to double vision.

There are many different types of contact lenses and manufacturers. Generically speaking, there are three types of contact lenses that predominate the field: soft, gas permeable hard, and scleral lenses.

Before we discuss the different types of contact lenses, it's super important to go over the caring of the lenses, which includes how to put them in and how to take them out. What's really important is patient hygiene. Patients must make sure their hands are clean and that the case they're storing the lenses in is clean.

One last important subject regarding contact lenses are the solutions patients use to clean and sterilize the lenses. I have seen patients suffer from significant discomfort from contact lenses because they're allergic to a particular brand of solution. This is not extremely common, but I have seen patients who have almost failed with contact lenses become extremely satisfied with them just by changing the solutions they are using. One last note about solutions is some of the care kits patients use utilize hydrogen peroxide for cleaning. Generally speaking, hydrogen peroxide needs to be neutralized before it goes into the eye. If it isn't, this leads to extreme discomfort and a trip to the eye doctor.

SOFT CONTACT LENSES

Let's start with soft contact lenses since this is what most patients are fitted with today. I am also going to start with what is known as a spherical lens. This is a lens prescribed for a patient who has minimal or no astigmatism. For the most part, they're comfortable and the vision they deliver when appropriately prescribed is good. There are several different brands. Each doctor usually has a brand that they start out with when fitting a patient. What's important to know is that there is no one lens out there that's the best for everyone. If the first choice doesn't give good vision, we check to see if the prescription is optimal before we go to another brand. If everything looks good with the lens we usually have the patient wear it for a week or two and come back to make sure it's fitting well.

Most soft contact lenses are on a frequent replacement basis. Some lenses are replaced monthly, or every two to three weeks and some are replaced every day. The modality results from a discussion between the doctor and the patient. Sometimes, patients may over wear their lenses including sleeping in them for long periods of time. Some lenses are approved for sleeping in but that doesn't mean each patient is capable of sleeping in them.

The second type of soft contact lens is the lens for astigmatism. This is called a toric lens. These are more difficult to fit. The lens has to rotate correctly in the eye for the patient to see well. The way it rotates is that one edge of the lens is thicker. For a few patients, this leads to some discomfort. The designs of these lenses are getting better all the time. Even in cases where it was difficult to fit a patient with a toric contact lens years ago, it's much easier to get the desired result today. If the astigmatism of the patient is very high we may need to fit a rigid, gas permeable lens.

The third type of soft contact lens that has really improved in quality is the multifocal contact lens. More and more patients are becoming successful wearers of these lenses and it has made a big difference in their lifestyle. Before these were developed, if a patient was in their forties or older, the only way they could see close-up was to wear reading glasses over their contact lenses or wear one contact lens for reading and one contact lens for distance which is called monovision (by the way, this monovision seldom works with glasses).

What is great about these lenses is that when they work, the patient can look up and down, left and right, without having to adjust their neck. I have had a tennis player and golfer respond enthusiastically to the use of multifocal contact lenses and their performance in their respective sport. Generally speaking, you can't play these sports with bifocal spectacle lenses.

GAS PERMEABLE LENSES

Rigid gas permeable lenses are hard (not soft) and generally a lot smaller than soft lenses. For these two reasons, when they're initially fitted, the patient feels more discomfort. Generally speaking, the vision with rigid gas permeable is very good. There are certain situations where you need to fit a rigid gas permeable lens for the patient to see. There are some corneal conditions where the patient could only see effectively with rigid gas permeables. One such condition is keratoconus. Keratoconus is a progressive, degenerative thinning of the cornea. As the condition progresses, the ability for the patient to see clearly out of glasses or soft contact lenses diminishes. These gas permeable lenses for keratoconus can be difficult to fit, so in most cases, I will refer any patients having the condition to specialists.

I mentioned earlier about scleral lenses. These are rigid gas permeable lenses that are a lot larger in nature and prescribed to individuals who have significant corneal problems. When I find a patient who has a condition that can benefit from these lenses, I refer them to a doctor who is skilled in fitting these lenses.

CONTACT LENS SAFETY

Contact lenses are generally safe to wear. However, I have seen some very serious eye infections result from them. This could result from over wearing contacts or not cleaning them correctly.

One of the more serious conditions occurring with contact lenses is the development of a corneal ulcer. This is a very serious infection which, if left untreated, can lead to a serious loss of vision. This is particularly true if the ulcer is located in the center of the cornea. In most cases, the ulcer generally resolves well with prescribed medication.

Another problem that can result from overwear of contact lenses is a condition called neovascularization. This is the formation of new blood vessels growing into the cornea (where there shouldn't be any blood vessels). Sometimes if the patient has this situation, they have to significantly reduce the wearing of the contact lenses and possibly start a regimen of medication to help alleviate this situation.

One other condition that has its roots from wearing contact lenses is giant papillary conjunctivitis (GPC). This is where there is inflammation under the upper lids of the patient. As the patient wears their contact lenses, the inflammation increases. This condition usually leads to discomfort while wearing contact lenses with the lenses getting foggy. Also with this condition, the contact tends to move quite a bit with each blink. I don't see this condition nearly as much now due to the use of disposable contact lenses.

When I find this condition, we sometimes have the patient stop wearing contact lenses for a while, and we begin administering medication, usually in the form of an anti-inflammatory. We also suggest that the patient start wearing daily contact lenses where each pair is thrown away after one day of use. This condition is sometimes very difficult to treat.

There are certainly more complications from contact lenses that exist but I wanted to describe the three main ones. What's important is that the contact lens wearer should be seen by their eye doctor every so often (as decided by the eye doctor) to help avoid any of the above situations.

Systemic disease and its Effect on the Eye.

DIABETES

Let's start with the biggie: diabetes. Diabetes is one of those diseases that has a tremendous impact on vision in various ways. There have been several times that patients have come into my office complaining of vision that has rapidly changed. Sometimes this could be that the patient started with very blurred distant vision and all of a sudden they see clearly without their glasses. This constitutes an immediate referral to their primary care physician to see if there's any systemic condition causing this change. Most of the time this is where the initial diagnosis of diabetes takes place.

The problem in prescribing glasses for these individuals is that by the time this patient receives their glasses, the prescription could change. In fact, the prescription can change several times until the sugar levels in the blood have stabilized. I prescribe disposable contact lenses to these patients. If the patient's eyes are constantly changing, you can change the contact lens prescription without any material costs. Also, there have been situations where an established diabetic patient will have a significant change in prescription over a short period, and we'll have to refer them back to their primary care physician to check their sugar levels.

The long-term effects of uncontrolled diabetes are a lot more serious. Three eye conditions can result from diabetes: cataracts, glaucoma, and retinopathy.

Changes in the sugar levels could affect the lens of the eye. This could cause a change in the prescription of the patient as described above. Also, the changes in the lens of the eye can cause a change where opacification occurs. This means that no matter what lens is prescribed for the patient, the patient will not be able to see clearly. If this progresses to a point where the best-corrected vision is unacceptable to the patient, cataract surgery may be performed where the lens of the eye is removed and replaced with an artificial lens. Even though no surgery is routine, this operation is relatively safe, and the outcome for some of the patients is literally miraculous with the improvement in vision being huge.

Long-term or uncontrolled diabetes can also cause glaucoma. Generally speaking, this is where the pressure of the eye increases, affecting the nerves of the eye and actually causing their death. One mechanism for the development of glaucoma is by a process called neovascularization. This is where new blood vessels form. These blood vessels sometimes grow where the fluid of the eye drains. In so doing, they keep the fluid in the eye from draining and therefore this can cause a spike in the pressure of the eye.

One of the most devastating effects of long-term or uncontrolled diabetes occurs in the retina of the eye, changes in the blood vessels (vasculature). This could cause bleeding in the back of the eye. This bleeding can severely affect one's vision. This is what is referred to as diabetic retinopathy. Getting one's sugar under control through diet and exercise can help keep this condition in check or keep it from progressing as rapidly. One new development over the last several years are drugs that are injected into the eye, which keeps the bleeding under control. In fact, in some cases, these drugs can actually restore some of the lost vision the patient has incurred.

HYPERTENSION

Uncontrolled hypertension can also lead to severe changes in the eye. Again, lifestyle changes can help keep retinopathy from occurring.

CHOLESTEROL AND TRIGLYCERIDES

High cholesterol or triglycerides can have an effect on vision. If a small plaque (an embolus) breaks off and travels to the eye through the arteries, this can cause a blockage of blood and can lead to partial blindness or even total blindness of the eye. This is because the area of the retina being served by those blood vessels isn't receiving any nutrients or oxygen. Also, a blockage of the carotid artery can lead to loss of vision for the same reason—no blood being able to travel to the eye.

CANCER AND AUTOIMMUNE DISEASES

When a patient has been diagnosed with and is being treated for cancer, it is important to thoroughly examine the back of the eye. There have been situations where the cancer has metastasized to the eye. In the early stages of the disease, the cancer in the eye can be treated. However, if the cancer is widespread within the eye, the eye may need to be removed (enucleated).

Separate from this type of cancer which can form in the back of the eye, there are various forms of skin cancer that can form on the lids. In the early stages, this can be treated. However, if it is left untreated, this cancer can spread to other parts of the body.

An autoimmune disease is where the body's immune system goes "haywire." Here the immune system views different tissues or organs within the body as "foreign" and attacks them. This could lead to inflammation in parts of the eye. Some of these diseases can cause a proliferation of white blood cells to congregate within the eye severely affecting vision. An additional problem occurs in actually treating the condition. Two medications that come to mind are steroids and hydroxychloroquine (Plaquenil). Steroids, when used to treat conditions within the body or the eye, can lead to glaucoma or cataracts in certain people. Plaquenil can cause changes in the part of the retina called the macula. This can lead to a loss of vision. This is why when doctors prescribe these medications, they have to make sure their patients are having their eyes examined on a regular basis. Of course, these are not the only medications that can cause problems with the eyes.

DISEASES WITHIN THE BRAIN

As I discussed earlier, diseases within the brain can cause changes in one's vision. An **aneurysm** in the brain can blur one's vision or cause a loss of periphery. This is before it ruptures. If it ruptures, it can cause death. A tumor can do the same.

The topic of **concussions** has been given a lot of attention lately, especially regarding sports. Double vision or blurred vision could certainly be due to a concussion. In addition to findings regarding mental status, observing one's pupils with regards to concussions is paramount. Are the pupils reacting normally to light? Is there a difference in the size of the pupils where none existed before? Realize there are other etiologies for defective pupillary findings.

Thyroid problems can lead to dryness of the eye which can lead to discomfort as well as blurred or double vision.

This above area of vision care is nowhere complete, but I wanted to cover some of the major diseases and their consequences.

EYE VITAMINS

One last area I briefly want to discuss is eye vitamins. There are studies that show the importance of certain vitamins regarding eye health, particularly the macula part of the retina. Two of them come to mind, lutein, and zeaxanthin. Lutein is generally found in deep, leafy green vegetables such as kale and spinach. Zeaxanthin is found in certain berries and perhaps peppers. Of course, there are supplements over the counter that contain these vitamins. These vitamins can certainly help prevent or slow the process of macular degeneration, a disease where the patient slowly loses their central vision.

One of the most important responsibilities I have as a clinician is the immediate referral to the appropriate health care professional who can best take care of these patients.

LOW VISION

Low vision is an area of optometry where patients are not capable of clear vision with glasses or contact lenses. Many times these individuals cannot see the big "E" on the chart even with conventional glasses or contact lenses. This could be due to a systemic disease or injury. The technology to have these individuals see and lead a relatively normal life has increased tremendously. This is why when I see any of these patients in the office, I refer them to the appropriate specialist.

VISION TRAINING

This is an area of optometry that is very dear to me. As I said earlier, my education included a very strong training in behavioral vision. Vision training is a huge part of behavioral optometry.

Part of vision training works with patients whose eyes are not straight. It also works with individuals, especially young kids, who are not capable of clear vision in one of their eyes. This condition defines amblyopia. In these cases, disease or injury has to be ruled out. In many cases, this condition developed pretty close to birth. As stated earlier, good binocular vision is a very important skill. It's important in learning, viewing near material like books, desktops and laptops, and all digital devices, including cell phones.

Good visual skills are also extremely important when it comes to education. Clear vision, of course, is important. Being able to track and not lose one's place while reading is essential. Many different types of visual skills are involved in education. These skills are sometimes enhanced by having a prescription designed particularly for near. Other visual skills needed for learning include aiming and focusing as well as being able to sustain close-up vision. There are other areas of vision development which deal with left-right awareness as well as mind and body development that are also involved with learning.

Binocularity is also paramount in sports. Think of the skills involved in performing any sport. Of course one has to be able to see clearly. Let's look at some of the other visual skills that one has to perform well: being able to have good peripheral vision and not have it tunnel down when you're under stress; being able to focus and aim your eyes efficiently so you can track a moving object; having good depth perception, judging how far away an object is from you while it's moving; being able to momentarily take your eye off the ball and being able to pick it up again. All of these skills are critical in most sports.

These skills could be enhanced significantly with vision training. As one approaches the professional level in any sport, any incremental improvement in one's skills, including vision, could have a tremendous effect on one's performance.

E-SPORTS

Over the last few months, I've come across patients who were involved with video streaming and competing in games digitally while viewing a monitor. This is generally referred to as E-sports. What an unbelievably tremendous area for optometry to get involved with. What a hugely competitive and visually stressful sport this is. There are colleges who are actually giving scholarships for Esports performance. There are actually teams and leagues being formed competing worldwide and the prize money is astounding. There are professional sports figures and teams (such as from the National Basketball Association) who are sponsoring and backing individuals and teams involved with E-Sports. Spectators view these competitions as if they're watching football or baseball with announcers calling the action.

The number of hours these individuals are on the screen as well as their intensity could very well be affecting their vision. Just as important is how their play could be improved with appropriate lenses for the display, as well as vision training to improve the necessary hand-eye coordination and vision skills necessary to maximize their results. Other factors that are also very important regarding the area of E-Sports is possible filtering out of blue light and vitamins that help protect the back of the eye from deleterious effects of the light emitted from the screen.

Studies have shown that enhancing and protecting the pigment in the macula and back of the eye through specific vitamins (as discussed earlier regarding macular degeneration) could very well improve the performance of these players.

One last area I want to cover is dry eye. Does the patient blink enough and is the dry eye significant enough to affect the performance of these players? There are various ways to help improve the comfort level and performance of an individual suffering from dry eye. This could include something as simple as over the counter artificial tears, prescription eye drops, punctal plugs (you can Google this term), vitamins containing omega-3, or even something as simple as blinking more.

Advances in the field of eye care have been huge.

I have been practicing optometry since 1981. Advances in my profession have been huge, covering a multitude of areas of patient care. Advances in lenses, contact lenses, treatment of diseases, surgeries, and instrumentation have certainly led to great outcomes in patient care.

There has been a substantial improvement in the lenses that patients order for their spectacles. This change has led to lenses being thinner with less distortion. I'd like to discuss some of these lenses below.

POLYCARBONATE LENSES

Over the years, polycarbonate lenses have become the standard for safety. They are mandated for all individuals under eighteen years old. They are extremely resistant to shattering while still being thin. In higher prescriptions, however, some patients feel they have some distortion to their vision. To fix this, high index plastic is a thinner material that is safe and has less distortion but is not quite as shatter-resistant as polycarbonate lenses.

PROGRESSIVE ADDITION LENSES

Progressive addition lenses are multifocal lenses without the line. The challenge with these kinds of lenses is to give a maximal area for reading while reducing peripheral distortion. Unfortunately, unless you've worn these lenses before, you probably will not understand what I'm talking about. The lens manufacturers have been able to improve the quality of these lenses quite dramatically over the years. Now there are progressive addition lenses that are quite specific for those patients who are sitting in front of a desktop monitor.

ANTI-REFLECTIVE COATING

Anti-reflective lenses have been around for decades. Anti-reflective lenses serve two purposes. The first one is cosmetic. When you wear these lenses they appear a lot more invisible to people who are looking at you, almost as if there is no lens in the frame. The second advantage is what the wearer sees. Basically what the patient is looking at appears clearer and there is a lot less glare and reflection with these lenses. This is particularly true while driving at night.

When anti-reflective lenses first came out, they scratched and smeared really easily. Over the years these problems have been reduced but not totally eliminated. In my opinion, for the most part, the positives about these lenses far outweigh the negatives.

BLUE LIGHT

A recent advancement over the years has been the development that helps to block blue light. This is particularly important for patients who are viewing monitors or digital devices. It has been shown that viewing digital devices before one goes to bed may interfere with one's sleep. Research is showing that this blue light might simulate daylight, which will suppress melatonin, which in turn can interfere with one's sleep. There is also debate about whether this light is harmful to the eye. There are lenses now being made by manufacturers that appear clear but significantly reduce this blue light. One very important point to consider is that if discerning various colors on your screen (for example being able to tell a light green from a slightly darker green) is important at the task at hand, this blue-blocking lens may interfere with this ability and therefore should not be used. It is important to note that some of the manufacturers of screens and devices are developing systems to automatically reduce this blue light when engaged.

Correcting one's vision without the use of glasses or contact lenses.

There are contact lenses that are used to help correct nearsightedness and astigmatism. The procedure is called orthokeratology where a patient will wear gas permeable hard contact lenses while they sleep which helps mold the cornea thusly changing the prescription. This allows the patient to see clearly during the day without glasses or contact lenses. Even though this is still performed by eye care professionals, most patients opt for a surgical procedure that helps reduce or eliminate the need for glasses or contact lenses.

The first major procedure to help correct a patient's prescription was called radial keratotomy. This was where radial cuts were administered into the cornea helping to change the cornea's shape, thus changing the prescription. There was some success with the procedure, but it was far from the success that is achieved today through the use of laser. As an optometrist, I have seen some major problems with some of my patients who have had radial keratotomy. For the most part, this procedure has not been performed to any great extent since the mid-late 1990s, I have seen patients coming into the office who have had this procedure. Realize these patients had the procedure over twenty years ago.

The problem with many of these patients is that their prescription has changed significantly from the time they originally had the surgery. Sometimes the cornea is so distorted that no matter what prescription we come up with, the patient can't see clearly. There is one more very important finding.

When the cornea is cut, the cornea is left weak. This is important because the shape of the cornea can be more easily changed than it was before the surgery was performed. As stated earlier, as the cornea changes shape, the prescription will change. It's important to realize that the internal pressure of the eye changes throughout the day. This is normal. When the cornea is at normal strength, the corneal shape will not vary with the change in pressure. However, in some cases of radial keratotomy, I have seen a patient's prescription change depending on the time of day, most likely due to the change of shape of the cornea.

Another important point is that many of the patients who have had the surgery are now ready to have cataract surgery. In some cases, it is more difficult to get as accurate an outcome for the cataract surgery if the patient has had radial keratotomy before.

LASER SURGERY

The use of laser over the years has dramatically improved the success of refractive surgery. Again this surgery helps to reduce or eliminate the need for a patient to wear glasses or contact lenses to see clearly. Generically speaking, two of the main types of laser surgery are referred to as LASIK or PRK.

With PRK, the laser is applied to the front surface of the cornea. This generally involves some pain and a longer time for the eye to heal and achieve clarity.

The other technique, LASIK, generally creates a flap where the laser is applied to an inner layer of the cornea and then the flap is laid back. Generally, this surgery has a quicker healing period with little or no pain.

Ideally, the surgery can correct one's vision better than glasses or contact lenses can. Measuring one's corneal health as well as thickness is critical. If the cornea is thin, PRK is generally performed. If the cornea is not healthy, neither of these surgeries is available.

An important point to cover is surgery for the patient over forty who generally has a different prescription for reading as compared to distance. Ways of dealing with this include a surgery where both eyes are corrected for distance and the patient will then have to wear reading glasses for close-up. Another option is to correct one eye for reading and one eye for distance. Quite often a patient will have experienced this before considering surgery by having worn contact lenses where one eye was fitted for reading while the other eye was fitted for distance.

Two other types of surgery can be performed on the cornea. With corneal Inlays, a piece of plastic is inserted into the layers of the cornea to help the patient see better close-up. Generally, this is done on one eye. Another type of corneal surgery generally performed is Intacs. This is generally performed on patients who don't have a high prescription. I have come across fewer patients who have had these surgeries recently.

Other forms of refractive surgery follow the same surgery as someone who had cataracts. In this case, the patient's lens is removed and a new one is inserted. The technology behind these lenses, intraocular lenses, is ever increasing. It used to be that these lenses would only correct for one distance (most times distance). They now have intraocular lenses that could give you correction for reading and distance. Sometimes with these specific lenses, there is some compromise in the near vision and sometimes the distance. A detailed questionnaire of the patient's work habits and visual demands, including how far away the reading material is from the patient should be administered.

One other type of surgery to help correct one's vision is by implanting a lens in front of or behind the pupil. There are advantages and disadvantages to this type of surgery that I will not go into here.

EYE HEALTH

Other advances in the eye-care field center around the health of the eye.

There are conditions that exist within the eye starting with the front surface of the eye (the cornea) going all the way to the back of the eye. Even though the following isn't exhaustive, the material is informative.

CORNEA

Let's start with the cornea. There are conditions that lead to a breakdown of the cornea. Some are pathological due to bacteria, viruses or fungal conditions. Many of these can be dealt with successfully with medications. However, if the pathological condition gets out of hand and the medications are ineffective, in extreme situations, a corneal transplant must be performed. The procedure for this surgery over the years has become less invasive and has become a lot more easily tolerated by the patient.

There are corneal conditions, some of which are genetic in nature. I want to touch on one, keratoconus. This is a condition where the cornea begins to thin and becomes cone-shaped. The patent will first notice that no matter what glasses they're wearing, they won't be able to see clearly. Generally, these patients are fit with gas permeable hard contact lenses so they can see. The problem with these is that, for some patients, the discomfort in wearing these lenses is unbearable. In some cases, over the years, the cornea will thin to such a degree that the only way to deal with the condition is replacing the cornea (as described above).

There is a relatively new procedure being performed on these patients to keep the cornea from thinning. It is called Corneal Cross Linking. Here, a specific chemical is combined with ultraviolet light helping to strengthen the cornea. This condition is usually performed with patients in their twenties and thirties. It has been met with success.

LENSES AND CATARACTS

Going further back into the eye we'll be dealing with conditions of the lens of the eye. In this case, we're discussing cataracts. Almost everyone develops cataracts as they age and generally, they need to be removed. The time for removal is generally when the patient is in their seventies to eighties. Cataract surgery has advanced tremendously over the years so that most patients have excellent vision after the surgery (barring any problems that already exist with the retina). As alluded to above, some of the advances in cataract surgery deal with the types of lenses that are inserted into the eye.

There have been advances with what is described as a multifocal intraocular lens. This allows for distance and near viewing. For some patients, there is some compromise in the near vision. Careful questioning of the patient's near visual demands, such as whether the patient does most of their reading at sixteen inches or twenty-two inches is critical in prescribing the appropriate lens. The most recent development is that there are intraocular lenses that are multifocal and correct for astigmatism. Keep in mind, however, that some patients handle one eye for reading and one eye for distance quite well.

THE RETINA

We have discussed various changes that occur in the retina due to disease, genetics, and aging. The technology that helps us diagnose problems occurring in the retina has tremendously increased over the years. We're able to measure subtle changes in the retina that the human eye has no way of seeing. I just want to cover two such diseases.

One deals with glaucoma. Glaucoma generally deals with the dying of nerves generally related to the pressure of the eye. Instrumentation allows us to monitor the health of the nerve layers in the retina which can help us better diagnose and treat the patient over time. The other diagnosis using this instrumentation is to study the health of the retina as a whole, particularly the macula (the central area of the retina), which, when affected, could significantly affect the patient's ability to see clearly.

There are books written solely about the retina—the area of the eye where light comes to a focus—sort of like the screen of the eye. In many cases when there is damage to the retina, there's very little that can be done to help correct the patient's vision. There are many ways the retina can be damaged. I'm going to cover a few of them and then go over what can be done to help correct the situation.

I want to start with the conditions of the retina that develop because of systemic diseases. The main disease I want to discuss is diabetes. As discussed previously, the effects that diabetes has on the eye are tremendous. First off, when a patient (even before they've been diagnosed with diabetes) notices a sudden change in vision along with extreme thirst, chances are the patient's sugar has spiked. Generally speaking, if the sugar is dealt with so it achieves a normal blood level, the vision will go back to where it was before the sugar spiked.

The main problem with diabetes and to a significant degree, high blood pressure, is the changes that occur with the retina. The better the patient takes care of themselves, the longer it takes for changes to occur in the retina. The term that applies to the retina is retinopathy. Due to the pathology of diabetes, the retina can be deprived of oxygen. The most important change that occurs is neovascularization, the formation of new blood vessels. These blood vessels are not normal in structure. They are weak and more importantly, they could leak blood. In so doing they could blur one's vision. This is one of the forms of macular degeneration that is called wet macular degeneration. This used to be a situation where the patient would lose their central vision and there wasn't anything that could be done.

However, in the last several years, there has been a new type of drug developed that helps to limit the growth of these defective blood vessels. The type of drug is called 'anti-vegf.' By eliminating these blood vessels, there is less blood and fluid floating around freely in the retina. Not only has this drug kept the patients from getting worse, but in some cases, it has also helped restore some of the lost vision. For some patients, this has almost been a miracle.

Another problem with the formation of these blood vessels is the spiking of pressure in the eye. As stated earlier, the mechanism of this is the formation of these blood vessels in the area of the eye which deals with the exit of fluid. The formation of these blood vessels keeps the fluid of the eye from draining effectively. This is what causes the spiking of pressure.

One last development I want to discuss is developments in the field of treating glaucoma. There are new medications developed which help to control the pressure of the eye. Just as important, there are new surgical techniques being developed that cause little damage to the eye (minimally invasive) and control the pressure.

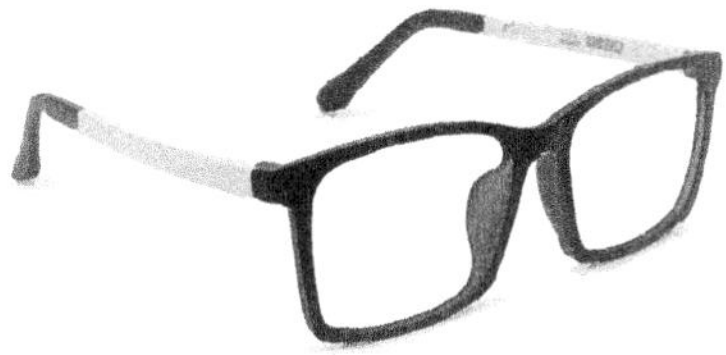

PART 3: MY PRACTICE IN 2019

As stated earlier, I graduated from optometry school in May 1981. I worked for other optometrists until 1989 when I opened my own practice. I feel so blessed that I am in my own practice. My passion for practicing optometry has grown over the years. With the proliferation of digital devices over the years, the need for my services has grown exponentially. When I first opened my practice in the spring of 1989, I made a ton of mistakes. Despite the many ups and downs concerning my practice, one thing is for certain—I always enjoyed working with patients! I really love the field of optometry.

Over the last several years, my practice has really begun to take off. I am fortunate that I have a really great staff. I am not a detail person when it comes to the running of a business but the staff backs me up. As stated earlier, my strengths lie in my clinical skills, my passion for the profession, and my ability to market the practice.

Over the last couple of years, I hired an individual to do my social media. I know what I want to say and video and I will go over later in the book the networks I am on. I generally need help in posting my information. She also keeps track of my engagement of individuals on the various sites. I know I need help with this but I really want to try to "Crush" this. Of course, this term I attribute to Gary Vaynerchuck (Gary Vee) and his book, *Crushing It.*

These are great times. When it comes to promoting yourself, the world is limitless. I realize that I am just scratching the surface, but my enthusiasm for getting my message out about not only optometry but also personal development is growing and I am hoping that it continues to grow exponentially. Just writing this book is an example of how much easier it is to publish now compared to years ago.

MY INSPIRATION

One of the books I have read which had a tremendous impact on my practice and life in general is Dale Carnegie's *How to Win Friends and Influence People.* I must have read this book at least ten times. It's as applicable today as when it was written over eighty years ago. The ability to deal with people effectively, making them feel comfortable and trusting, is such an important part of one's business success as well as life in general. Empathy, which is covered in this book as well as by Gary Vee, is so important. Trying to put yourself in another individual's place or situation is paramount in dealing with people.

The journey (as described in many of Gary Vee's publishings) to a successful practice has been difficult at times and so rewarding at other times. I feel so blessed professionally and personally. And the greatest part is that the journey is far from over. I have said to numerous family members and friends that I'll be doing things in a couple of years, and I really don't know what they are right now. One year ago, I had no idea that I would be writing a book. I attended a social media conference in San Diego in February 2018, and there was a course in self-publishing.

I also feel my self-awareness (another term brought out by Gary Vee) has been growing exponentially. I am really excited about how my practice has developed over the last few years as has my standing in the business community and professional community. I also feel really great about how my relationships with my extended family members have grown. I believe it's because I really believe I have a positive spirit.

I truly believe this positivity has helped lead to the success of my practice. From the greeting when the patient first enters the office (either by my staff or me) to the time the patient leaves, the patient is surrounded by positive, upbeat individuals.

DEVELOPING LEGACY AND BRAND

It is really neat that I have seen some of my patients beginning as kids growing up and now I see their children. It's really a great feeling having developed a feeling of trust among these patients and the ones who I am currently seeing. When working with patients, listening to their symptoms and problems concerning their vision is paramount. Much of this is covered in taking a good case history. I feel particularly fortunate that I am independent of anyone telling me how to examine a patient or how much time to devote to a patient. Being independent also allows me to delegate areas of my practice to my staff. Believe me, in certain cases, my staff is better than I am in running certain parts of my practice. What's also important is I know there are various areas of eye care where there are professionals better equipped and educated to work with certain types of vision problems. When I get patients with needs outside my realm of practice, I always refer them to another professional.

I read and listen to books and online material about business development. One of the areas frequently covered is developing one's brand. I really feel that I have done that. Except in rare circumstances, when a patient makes an appointment in my practice they know they're going to see me. So what is my brand? Patient interest and community involvement.

PATIENT INTEREST

First of all, it is actually developing a sincere interest in the patient's visual system as well as the total patient. It is asking questions of the patient to see what type of problems they're having visually, their interests in work, education, and play. Then, after examining the patient, it involves coming up with a plan—whether it be with glasses, contact lenses, vision training, referral to an outside specialist, or a combination of the above. What's important is that I listen to what the patient wants and then present options to the patient they might not have thought of. This conversation takes time and it isn't rushed. Sometimes it's fairly straightforward and sometimes we have to go into detail of a plan that the patient never heard of before.

Part of my brand is that I have a lot of passion when it comes to delivering care. One small example of this occurs when a patient is trying on glasses. If a patient has an extreme prescription, they might not be able to see the glasses they're trying on. In that situation, we'll ask the patient if they want me to place a pair of contacts on their eyes. Of course, there isn't any obligation in getting contacts but at least they can see what they're trying on. Just a side note, some of these patients have never worn contacts and this is the first time they can see clearly without glasses. Occasionally, this is a big deal for the patient.

My goal with my patients is to put myself in their place and figure out how I would like to be professionally treated. Just talking to a patient about their interests, whether visual or life in general, is important. You see, vision is a very emotional sense and when we have the potential to improve it or introduce something to the patient that they have never been shown, it is a really big deal for the patient. Here is a great example. I have had several patients whose vision is a lot worse in one eye than the other eye. Not only that, the eye with the worse prescription isn't able to see, even with the glasses. So in many cases, the patient doesn't wear any glasses and just ignores the worse eye. Keep in mind in many cases the eye is healthy but the patient, no matter what, can't make out any letters on the eye chart. However, the patient could very well have good peripheral vision. With a big prescription difference between the two eyes, if you put glasses on the patient which sit around a half-inch from the eyes, the patient might see distorted or double or ignore the image from the eye as the image size between the two eyes is different.

I know I have stated this earlier but it bears repeating. I have put contact lenses on these patients and all of a sudden they now have vision on that side where they never had it before. Keep in mind that the patient might not be able to see the letters on the eye chart but they may have vision on that side for the first time.

Also, they may notice that the world jumps into depth. The look on these patients' faces is so rewarding to me. Also, keep in mind that wearing the contact lens may have no effect on the patient. As I am writing this, I am realizing another important point. If a patient has only one functional eye, they should be wearing a pair of shatter-resistant glasses (with a prescription or not) to protect the eyes, particularly the eye that sees well.

COMMUNITY INVOLVEMENT

As I've said earlier, I am very involved with the local chambers of commerce in my community. I have given discussions on vision to these groups. I have also answered any personal vision questions the members may have. I have belonged to the Rancho Cucamonga Chamber of Commerce since 1989, ever since I opened my private practice. For the most part, I am the only optometrist that shows up to some of the chambers I belong to.

I really do enjoy discussing various aspects of life, especially with young individuals whom I run into. I'm sixty-two years old now. Physically, I'm in really good shape. I work out quite a bit at 24-Hour Fitness where I lift and really enjoy spinning. I am quite enthusiastic while working out, particularly in spin class, yelling a bit. It's really neat because quite a few of the members will ask me questions about their own visual situations or the situations of their friends or family members. Being part of the health care community, I feel it's important that I be in fairly good physical shape. I so enjoy talking about my profession with members and employees of the gym. I have actually gotten quite a few patients from these chats. On one occasion, I counseled an employee (also a student) who worked at the front desk at the gym. I asked her what career path she was heading for. She knew I was an optometrist and I did speak enthusiastically about the profession. After several of these discussions, she decided she wanted to become an optometrist. She was a really good student. I had her intern in my office for about 120 hours before she applied to optometry school. As it turned out, she was accepted. She graduated in 2015.

Another individual (at the front desk of the gym) and I got into a discussion, and I wound up giving her two books. The first one was *How to Win Friends and Influence People* and the second one was Gary Vaynerchuk's *Crushing It.* I feel the content in these two books is great.

A heartfelt moment for me was receiving a birthday card from a friend whom I met through the chamber. She thanked me for sharing my wisdom and stories and said I was the "patriarch of the community." That meant so much to me.

One of the neatest things was I would occasionally have my mother come into the office. As stated earlier, I would also bring her to many chamber events. I would also discuss her longevity, her kindness (sort of legacy and brand). Often my patients and members of the community would ask me how she was doing. She was such an ingratiating lady. When she passed on January 31, 2018, the beautiful words and thoughts my patients and the community shared were extremely heartfelt.

In closing, I believe that this quote from President Theodore Roosevelt describes how most people feel about those they encounter:

"Nobody cares how much you know until they know how much you care." I truly believe my staff and I live up to this quote.

INTERJECTING NEW YORK CITY

I'm originally from Long Island (Westbury). My love for New York City is great. Right now, I make three to four trips to The City a year. Whenever my patients tell me they're taking a trip to NYC, I go over with them places that they should visit. In fact, I give most of them my cell phone number so if they have any questions while there, they can call me. What's interesting is that everyone (and I really can't think of an exception) who has gone to NYC really loved it.

What the heck, I'll give a few points of interest in NYC that are not the typical tourist attractions.

Since I'm a Yankee fan. I'll start off with Yankee Stadium. Going to The Stadium only applies if you're there when the Yankees have a home game. If they're not home the Yankees have scheduled tours of the Stadium. I felt the tour of Wrigley Field (the Cubs home field in Chicago) was better. Here's an idea. If you go to a night game at the Stadium, arrive early and visit the Little Italy section of The Bronx. They have many wonderful restaurants there but one of my favorites is Emilia's. It's located around 187th Street and Arthur Avenue. It's difficult to get to as the closest subway is over a mile away. Uber might be a good way. The food is really great. After dinner, the owner will call for car service and they could drop you off at one of the subways that stop at Yankee Stadium (161st Street). Don't have the driver take you all the way up to the Stadium as the traffic is terrible. After the game, there are a few bars across the street that you can visit. My favorite is the Yankee Tavern on 161st St. Even if you don't drink, it's a great place to congregate after the game.

One of the things I most enjoy about the City is just walking. There are so many different types of walking tours. These tours include learning about different areas of NYC, food tours, and even the Gangster Tour.

If you would rather ride, there are different bus tours that you might want to investigate. One such tour is called "The Ride." Instead of me telling you about it, you can look it up on Google. I went on "The Ride" with my sister and I really enjoyed it.

There are a number of roof-top bars in NYC. One of my favorites because of its view is Ophelia's. It is located at First Avenue and 49th St. (actually Mitchell Place). I have been going there since 1980. It closed while the building was converted from a hotel to condominiums. The view is 360*. It's a great way to finish up an evening.

I really enjoy discussing these places with my patients. What's interesting is that my patients knowing I'm from N.Y. tell me about their trips there and usually tell me what a great time they had.

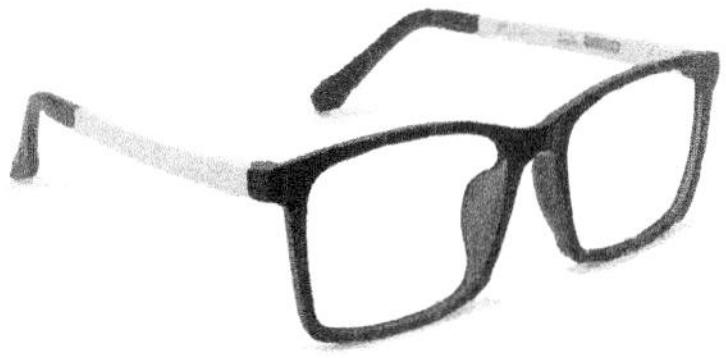

GLOSSARY OF TERMS

Amblyopia—Sometimes amblyopia is called lazy eye. Amblyopia is where one eye cannot see clearly even with glasses or contact lenses. One must rule out the disease of the eye. Generally, one thinks of amblyopia starting at a very young age. One reason amblyopia can occur is that an individual may have one eye with no prescription and the other eye has a very significant prescription. The individual "adapts" so that they only look out of the eye with little or no prescription and the vision in the eye having the high prescription doesn't develop. Sometimes patching the good eye and catching the amblyopia early and prescribing lenses or contact lenses can help

Aneurysm—A ballooning and weakened area of the artery.

Astigmatism—Literally means no point focus. If you have a significant amount of astigmatism and look at the letter "E," you may see the sideways lines clearer than the up and down line or visa versa.

Binocular Vision—Both eyes being able to aim and focus together so the individual sees one image. A person who has one eye that deviates in a direction different from the other eye does not have binocular vision

Blue filtered lenses—These are lenses that have a coating either on the surface or built in that helps protect the user from blue light. It has been shown that blue light could be harmful to various structures of the eye, particularly the macula (this term will be described further in the glossary). The blue filter will help to screen this light. Blue light has been shown to simulate daylight which suppresses melatonin within the body. If a digital device is used before someone goes to bed, it may keep them from sleeping. Also, it should be noted that some digital devices screen blue light on their own.

Cataract—A cataract is a clouding or opacification of the lens of the eye. It's generally, but not always, related to the age of the individual. Trauma or disease to the eye can also precipitate cataract formation. When the cataract causes a significant loss of clear vision, the lens can be removed and replaced with a plastic intraocular lens.

Cornea—The cornea is a tissue that's the most anterior surface of the eye. It controls a significant amount of how well an individual is able to see.

Corneal Cross-Linking—This is a procedure to help remedy keratoconus (discussed later in the glossary) by stabilizing the cornea.

Dry eye—This term relates to the front surface of the eye, particularly the cornea. There are three layers of fluids composing the tears, the mucin, the water, and the oily layers. If any of these layers become compromised, it could lead to dry eye. What's interesting is that a person could have an eye that excessively waters due to dryness.

E-Sports—These are massive competitions among individuals competing in video games. It has grown to such a tremendous level that some colleges are offering scholarships and professional sports teams like the New York Yankees are sponsoring individuals and teams involved with this.

Glaucoma—A disease process in the eye where the nerves receiving light in the back of the eye die. The general culprit for the disease is a rise in the fluid pressure within the eye. This is generally painless but can lead to a loss of peripheral vision first, then total vision if left untreated. Glaucoma is generally treated with drops, laser surgery, or insertion of a stint that helps to drain off the fluid and thusly lower the pressure.

Hemianopsia—This relates to a loss of half of an individual's peripheral vision. Generally, this is due to a disease process going on in the brain, a stroke, aneurysm, or a tumor.

Hyperopia—The individual has to use more effort to see close-up than far away (farsightedness).

Keratoconus—A weakening process of the cornea which leads to a thinning and distortion of the cornea. This usually leads to a loss of clear vision, even with glasses and contact lenses. Corneal cross-linking, as discussed earlier, is one technique to help arrest the weakening of the cornea and to help stabilize it.

LASIK (laser in situ keratomileuses)—This is a laser procedure performed on the cornea, which helps correct nearsightedness, farsightedness, and astigmatism.

Macula—The macula is the central part of the retina (discussed later in the glossary), which is the region of clearest vision. If there is a defect in this part of the retina, vision becomes significantly blurred.

Multifocal contact lenses—These are contact lenses, which help an individual see far and near, especially for those over forty who have presbyopia (described below).

Myopia (nearsightedness)—The individual is able to see better up close than far away.

Optic nerve—The visual signal is transmitted from the optic nerve which inserts in the back of the eye along a nerve pathway to the back of the brain in the area known as the visual cortex.

Polycarbonate lenses—These are lenses that are fitted into glasses. They're generally lighter in weight, have reduced thickness, and resist shattering if an object is to strike them. They're generally regarded as the standard of care for safety lenses, and lenses to be prescribed for children.

Presbyopia—As we age, the ability of the lens to change shape in the eye as we look at different distances diminishes. This usually starts to occur when the individual approaches forty years of age.

Prism—A prism is a lens that shifts the location of an object up, down, left, or right, depending on how it is positioned. It is generally prescribed to allow the eyes to work easier together.

Radial Keratotomy—This was one of the first procedures developed in the late 1970s and early 1980s, which actually used a blade to cut into the cornea to help improve one's vision. It has fallen out of favor with procedures such as LASIK as it's not nearly as precise and there are changes in vision that can occur later in life.

Retina—The retina is the back of the eye, generally regarded as the "screen" where the light focuses upon.

Retinopathy—This is where the retina is compromised by disease. Diabetes and hypertension are the two main culprits, but bacteria, fungus, viruses, and parasites could also wreak havoc with the retina.

Streff syndrome—This is like a spasming of the focusing system where the lens cannot relax focus. It leads to blurred vision. It is sometimes hard to diagnose as other conditions that can be pathological in nature must be ruled out first.

Visual Acuity—Visual acuity indicates how clearly one sees, generally measured at distance and sixteen inches. The term 20/20 means that a letter designed to be seen at 20 feet can be seen at 20 feet by the individual. An individual who has 20/400 at distance means an individual has to walk up to 20 feet to see a letter that normally is able to be seen at 400 feet.

Visual field testing—In obtaining a visual field, the individual is viewing a central target with one eye covered and their peripheral vision is measured. Then the other eye is tested. If there be a defect in the visual field, one must have further testing done by CT or MRI to determine the etiology of the defect.

Vision training—Generally speaking vision training is performed to help the eyes work better together. This applies to learning, work, and sports and E-Sports. The hope of vision training is to help the individual's performance in the above areas.

Vitamins—There is a lot of information regarding vitamins as they relate to the health of the eye. The two chief ingredients within these vitamins are lutein and zeaxanthin. The chief area where these vitamins help protect the eye is the macula.

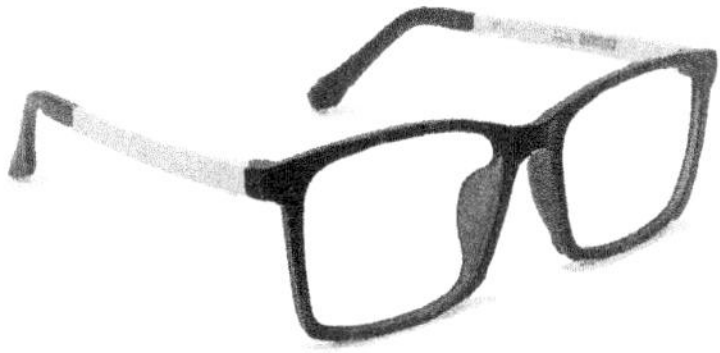

ABOUT THE AUTHOR

It's hard to believe Dr. Bob Rothbard has been practicing optometry for thirty-eight years. Getting into optometry school was difficult and stressful. One of his greatest sources of accomplishment was his acceptance letter to optometry school. He was blessed with parents who let him choose his profession and who gave their full support. They also supported his move to California from New York to establish his career.

Between Pacific University, College of Optometry, and a brief summer intern program at the State College of Optometry in New York City, he developed a model of behavioral vision that has served him well throughout his professional career. He looks at how vision affects many aspects of life, including work performance, education, and play, and how what you do in life affects your vision.

Now in his sixties, Dr. Bob is more excited about optometry than ever and finds great joy in his private practice and the staff and patients he works with daily. He also loves sharing his beliefs and knowledge about vision to the public via public speaking and social media. At this stage, Dr. Bob doesn't have any plans of retiring. Both the need for his services and the love from his patients makes it so easy to stay very involved with the practice.

Find Dr. Bob at:

LinkedIn: "Robert Rothbard."
Instagram: @ranchooptometric.
Twitter: @askdrbob and @BobRothbard
YouTube: "Robert Rothbard" and "Robert Rothbard, OD."
Facebook Fanpages: "Ranchoeyedoctor,"
PersonallyDevelopedSelf" and "NewYorkExperienced."

If you should need to contact him personally, please email: ranchooptometric@verizon.net.

Printed in Dunstable, United Kingdom

70367386R00061